HOME WORKOUTS

ANYONE | ANYTIME | ANYWHERE

FUN AND SIMPLE NO-EQUIPMENT HOME WORKOUTS TO HELP LOSE WEIGHT, BUILD MUSCLE AND ACHIEVE YOUR DREAM BODY

By

A.G. SCOTT

CONTENTS

This book is dedicated to the loving memory of A.A.N.

I love and miss you, and you are always in my thoughts.

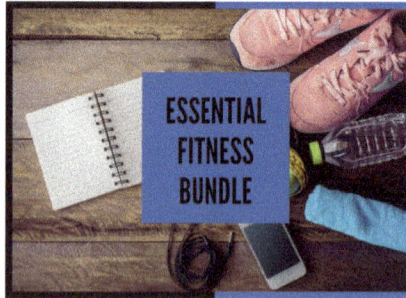

(Do NOT exercise without this...)

As a thank you for purchasing this book, I have thrown in a special gift for you. This bundle includes:

- An essential fitness checklist to ensure you have everything you need for your workout and where you can buy them for a great price
- 4 weeks' worth of exercise routines
- Two different types of personalisable fitness diary and a progress tracker to help you monitor your progress and track your success
- A weekly meal planner to help you organise what you'll be eating each day

The last thing I want is for your hard work to go to waste because you do not have the essentials. To receive your bundle, visit the link below:

https://agscott.activehosted.com/f/1

INTRODUCTION

E xercise. Whether you are a seasoned gym-goer or a bit of a gymaphobe, the power it holds to make you happier and healthier is probably no secret to you. In a perfect world, we would all have the motivation and time to exercise and go to the gym, but real life just isn't like that.

Sure, there are 24 hours in a day, but it often feels like less. We are all busy people, balancing our work lives with our home lives, and this becomes even more challenging when there are spouses, children, and pets to plan around. Understandably, exercise isn't always a priority and it can be difficult to squeeze it into your day.

Spending time in the gym can take a lot of time out of your day too. Let's say it takes you 15 minutes to get there, 60 minutes to do your routine and then 15 minutes to travel back home. That's 90 minutes out of your day (or 7.5 hours if you go five times a week) that you could spend doing other things such as enjoying quality time with your family, trying out a new hobby or even reading that new book you've heard so much about.

Fortunately, this book offers the perfect solution. In the chapters to come, I will talk you through exercises that will strengthen your muscles, improve your overall cardiovascular fitness and be a positive outlet for your everyday stress. As an added bonus, you can perform these exercises from the comfort of your own home with no need for any gym equipment. All you need is your body weight, gravity and around 20 to 30 minutes of free time.

My name is Archie; I am a medical student and I am interested in Sports Medicine and nutrition. I had been a regular gym-goer for many years and even used the occasional personal trainer to help me get in shape. However, this was expensive, and I struggled to fit the gym into my busy day-to-day schedule. I decided it was time to work out smarter instead of harder. I ended up terminating my gym membership and decided to pursue my fitness and body goals with home workouts instead.

My entire view on exercise has changed since I started home workouts, and I have been delighted with my progress. I continue to get fitter and I have more time throughout my week to focus on the other things in life I enjoy.

I decided to share my experience with my friends and family, and many of them started incorporating some home workouts into their daily routines. They too were very pleased with their results. They continually suggested that I write a book to help others reap the benefits too – so here it is mother! Working out doesn't need to be time-consuming, overly expensive, or keep you from enjoying the things you love. It should be a part of the day you look forward to and thanks to this book, that is what it will become.

These exercises are perfect for any fitness level

Regardless of your fitness level and experience, these workouts challenge you without leaving you feeling deflated. These exercises can be modified and altered to suit the fitness level you are at. You can easily add in extra repetitions, shorten the rest periods or incorporate additional movements to the exercises to push yourself further as your fitness and strength levels increase. Alternatively, there are ways to make the exercises easier to help ease you into them.

These exercises are perfect for burning fat

High-intensity interval training (HIIT) using your body weight is one of the best methods to burn fat because the body experiences the "afterburn" effect. This effect occurs when your body is working harder than normal to repay the oxygen debt that occurs during the workout in an effort to return itself to a normal resting state. In simple terms, your body keeps burning calories for hours after you have finished exercising because it is trying to restore balance. Studies have shown that the more intense your workout, the more calories you will burn and continue to burn for a longer period of time.

These exercises will improve your mental health

Exercise makes you feel good because it results in the release of endorphins. Endorphins help to relieve any underlying stress, naturally reduces blood pressure and makes you feel better about yourself and your surroundings, significantly helping to improve your mental health. People who exercise regularly can have lower chances of developing depression and anxiety, and studies have shown that the endorphins released during exercise can continue to be released for up to 24 hours after you have stopped exercising.

These exercises are convenient and space-efficient

Home workouts are very convenient and accessible. You don't need any gym equipment for these exercises, and they can easily be performed on a bedroom or living-room floor. All you need is a little bit of space and you can fit these exercises into your daily routine, whenever you have a bit of time. If you prefer to exercise in private, these exercises are perfectly suited for inside your house, or if you prefer the outdoors, your garden or the local park also work well.

These exercises are great for both cardio and strength training

Cardio isn't everyone's cup of tea. Not all of us enjoy going for 5-mile runs or swimming 400 meters early in the morning. Thankfully, these home workout exercises improve your cardiovascular fitness while also building the strength of your muscles. Bodyweight exercises such as push-ups and squats cause your heart rate to spike and adding in cardio exercises such as high knees and jumping jacks to your routines helps to keep the heart pumping harder for longer.

These exercises will build your core strength

Your core strength is more important to your body's wellbeing than most people realize. Your core is like Batman, the silent protector of Gotham, but one who doesn't get much credit. A strong core protects the spine and promotes strength in the muscles close to it, and bodyweight training is one of the best ways to improve your core strength because many of the exercises directly or indirectly target the body's core. These bodyweight exercises will not only improve your core strength, they will also improve your posture by strengthening your back muscles. Stronger back muscles will help prevent your shoulders from hunching forward and help to relieve any underlying back pain.

These exercises will improve your balance and flexibility

Some bodyweight exercises such as the single-leg reverse lunge are great for improving your balance as the movements help to develop your body awareness and control. Bodyweight exercises can also improve your flexibility, as they use the entire range of the joints, which helps ensure they are moving freely without restriction.

These exercises can help prevent injuries

Life can be unpredictable, and injuries can have a significant impact on day-to-day living. They can affect the body physically, preventing you from doing everyday activities such as washing and dressing independently, playing games with your children and enjoying your hobbies. They can also have a considerable effect on your mental health. It is imperative to ensure you train properly to avoid any injuries. Thankfully, workouts using your body weight are generally safer than free weight training, regardless of your age, fitness level, or prior exercise experience.

An added benefit of bodyweight exercise is that it can also reduce the risk of injuries occurring, especially exercises that target the core muscles. Stronger muscles are less likely to be injured, and it is no surprise that many athletes often bounce back relatively quickly after a muscular injury.

These exercises are enjoyable

It's no secret that traditional workouts can become dull and monotonous as time goes on as the lack of variety can turn exercise into a laborious chore. However, with bodyweight training, there are lots of different ways you can work out, and this variety helps to keep your workout routines fresh and enjoyable. You can even turn your workouts into a social event by gathering a group of friends together and performing these routines as a group.

You will see visible results

Training using your body weight is an effective (and free) method of achieving fast and visible results, as most of the exercises involve the use of compound movements. These movements employ the use of multiple muscle groups and use up more energy to do so, resulting in more calories being burned. Compound movements such as push-ups and squats are full-body exercises that involve several muscle groups all working at the same time. Research has shown that these types of movements are extremely effective for developing strength and muscle endurance while simultaneously burning unwanted body fat.

———

If you still aren't convinced, recent statistics have shown that approximately 62.5 million people had gym memberships in the United States in 2018. However, only about 18% of members attended the gym regularly.

With the average gym membership costing around $58 a month, 82% of members are paying for a service they don't consistently use. As each month passes, all that money adds up and becomes a significant amount at the end of the year – $696 annually. This isn't a trend isolated solely to the United States either; this is something that is happening globally. If you are one of those people, then it is time to stop spending your money on unused gym memberships and personal trainers and invest in this book to start improving your physical and mental health, save money and have more time to enjoy life.

With my help, you will be fully equipped with the knowledge to help you achieve your dream body. The information you're going to receive in this book will help you change the way you see exercise. Each chapter is tailored to target specific muscle groups, educate you on the anatomy of the muscles in each region and explain the benefits of each exercise. The proper techniques to adopt and common mistakes will also be detailed to help avoid any injuries and ensure you're getting the most out of your workout.

If you follow the training and the principles in this book, you will have taken the first step on your journey to achieving your dream body, all from the comfort of your own home. Putting off getting your health back on track shouldn't be delayed any longer. If you start today, think how much better you will look and feel in a month.

Medical Disclaimer

Before beginning any exercise or training program, it is strongly advised that you consult with your physician or primary care provider, as you should be in good physical health to participate in these exercises. Stick closely to the book and the techniques and ensure that you have dedicated enough time to warm up and cool down adequately.

This book describes the correct technique to use when performing each exercise, and there are proper and safe ways to do these exercises that will significantly reduce your risk of injury. However, when participating in any exercise or training routine, there is the possibility of physical injury. You may feel tired undergoing these exercises, and that is entirely normal. However, if you feel any unusual pain, please stop the activity immediately and seek medical help if you are concerned. If you are injured, do not attempt these exercises until you have fully recovered.

If you voluntarily engage in these exercises, you agree that you are doing so at your own risk, you will work to your own physical ability and not exceed your physical limits. You assume all risk of injury to yourself and agree to release and discharge the writer from any and all claims or causes of action, known or unknown, arising out of this book.

1

THE BASICS

B efore we get into the exercises, this chapter is going to explore some basic fundamentals that are important for every workout routine. These aspects are warming up, cooling down, the key principles of training and hydration.

Warming up and cooling down involves performing an activity/exercise at a slow, relaxed pace. Even though they may add a little bit of time to your workout, they are beneficial for your body and should never be overlooked.

WARMING UP

Warming up is often avoided because it adds extra time to your workouts. However, it doesn't need to take hours out of your day and even taking 5 minutes to warm up helps to ensure your body is better prepared for its workout.

Warming up is an essential part of your workout, and it typically involves a combination of some cardio and stretching exercises. These exercises help to raise your body temperature, slowly raise your heart rate and increase blood flow to the muscles, preparing your muscles and joints for the higher intensity exercises that are coming up. It can also reduce the likelihood of injuries occurring as warm muscles are far less likely to be injured than cold muscles.

It is important to use warm-up methods that target the same muscle groups you are planning on training as this will help prepare those muscles for the exercises to come. In the case of bodyweight exercises, the warm-up will involve the whole body as you are using several muscle groups during each exercise. There is no set rule on how to warm-up, but here is one of the most effective ways to do it:

1. Mini cardio exercises
2. Dynamic stretches

Mini Cardio Exercises

The mini cardio exercises help to raise your heart rate, increasing the blood flow to the muscles and warming them up. These exercises can be as simple as jogging or marching on the spot for a few minutes. Here are some mini cardio exercises to incorporate into your warm up:

- Jogging/marching on the spot
- High knees
- Star jumps
- Heel flicks/butt kicks

I would recommend spending 30-60 seconds on each exercise then moving on to the next one.

Dynamic Stretches

For years, static stretching, where you remain still and hold a stretch/pose for 10-30 seconds to lengthen the muscles, was one of the most popular methods to warm-up. However, dynamic stretching is the go-to method nowadays. Dynamic stretching involves actively moving your joints and muscles through a full range of motion.

These exercises can mimic the movements that you will be performing during the workout/activity, for example, performing arm circles if you are going to be swimming. Alternatively, these can simply be a series of movements to get your whole body ready for any type of exercise.

Dynamic stretches are beneficial for many reasons. They help to activate many muscles at the same time, help to improve your balance and coordination, and help to produce more heat in your body, ensuring you are ready for your exercise session.

However, it is important not to stretch when your body is cold because this can damage your muscle fibers. If you picture your muscles like a cold rubber band, they can't stretch as far when they are cold compared to when they are hot, so make sure to do your stretches after your mini cardio exercises. Since bodyweight training involves many muscle groups, your dynamic stretches should encompass all of these groups. Here are some dynamic stretches to do for your upper and lower body to help ensure you are fully prepared for your workouts.

Upper Body

- Wrist rotations – Stand upright and lift your arms straight out in front of you. Keep your arms still and start making circles with your wrists away from your body. Perform this movement for 15 to 30 seconds and then repeat this movement moving your wrists in the opposite direction.
- Arm rotations – Stand upright and raise your arms straight out to the side, so your body is in a T-shape. From here, start making small circles with your arms, gradually increasing the size of the circles as time goes on. Perform this movement for 30 to 60 seconds and then repeat the motion with your arms in the other direction.
- Arm hugs – Stand upright and raise your arms straight out to the side, so your body is in a T-shape. Bring your arms in and

wrap them around your chest, as if you are giving yourself a big hug, and then extend your arms out to the side again, moving them as far back as you can to help stretch the muscles in your chest. Repeat this movement for 30 to 60 seconds.

- Plank walkout – Stand upright with your arms by your side and then bend forward until your hands are flat on the ground in front of you, bending your knees slightly if you need to. From here, slowly walk your hands out in front of you, lowering your body into a high plank position, where your legs are straight out behind you, your back is straight, and your hands are shoulder-width apart. Perform a push-up (only if you want to) and then walk your hands back in towards your body and stand upright again. Perform this movement 10 times.

Lower Body

- Leg kicks with opposite arm reach – Stand to the left of a raised surface that you can rest your right hand on to keep you balanced, such as a table, chair or railing. Keep your back upright and lift your right leg off the ground, balancing on your left leg. Lift your right leg back behind your body, then swing it in front of you as high as you can in a kicking motion and reach for your toes with your left hand. Perform this movement 10 times before turning 180-degrees and performing 10 leg kicks with your left leg.
- Lunge with spinal twist – Stand upright with your hands by each side and lunge forward with your right leg. Try to lower yourself down until your right thigh is parallel to the ground with your right knee bent at 90-degrees and your left knee is hovering just above the ground. Don't let your right knee roll further forward than your toes. Once you are in the lunge position, twist your upper body to the right and then to the left. From here, push through your right foot and return to a

standing position. Repeat this movement 10 times, alternating between lunging with your left and right leg.

- Gate openers – Stand with your feet hip-width apart. Lift your right foot off the ground until your knee is in line with your right hip. From here, move your right knee out away from your body (like you are opening a gate) until it is pointing out to the side while simultaneously rotating your upper body as you perform this movement. Finally, place your right foot on the ground. Then, reverse this movement by lifting your right foot off the ground, raising your knee to hip height, bringing it back in towards your body then lowering your foot to the ground again. Perform this movement 10 times and then repeat with your other leg. You can hold on to a stable surface to help keep your balance if you need to.

- Ankle rotations – Stand with your feet hip-width apart and lift your right foot slightly off the ground, balancing on your left leg. Start rotating your right foot in clockwise circles for 15 to 30 seconds, then rotate your foot anticlockwise for 15 to 30 second. Repeat this movement with your left foot.

Now that you have finished your mini cardio exercises and dynamic stretches, you are ready to start your workout.

COOLING DOWN

Similar to warming up, cooling down is another important aspect of exercise that is neglected by many people. Micro-tears occur in the muscle fibers during exercise and this, combined with the production of lactic acid, are the main contributors to muscle stiffness. This feeling of stiffness and pain can carry on for several days and can result in delayed onset muscle soreness (DOMS). However, cool down exercises can help prevent this from happening or reduce the severity of DOMS.

Cooling down involves performing exercises at a slow and gentle pace, helping to gradually bring your body back into its resting state. It helps to slowly bring your heart rate, temperature and blood pressure down, break down the excess lactic acid that is produced during exercise and speeds up the healing process in your muscles.

Cooling down is a process that can be adapted according to personal preferences and the type of activities you have done. Similar to warming up, there is also no set way to cool-down, but here is one of the most effective ways to do it:

1. Light jog/slow walk
2. Static stretches

While dynamic stretches are beneficial when warming up, they shouldn't be used as a way to cool-down. Dynamic stretches raise your body temperature and therefore aren't useful when your aim is to slowly lower your temperature.

To cool down, start with a light jog or slow walk (either outside or on the spot) for 2 to 3 minutes. You want to keep moving to help reduce the amount of lactic acid that builds up. Then choose some static stretches from the list below, focusing on stretches which target the regions of the body you have exercised. As your muscles are warm and the blood flow to them has increased, you may notice that your muscles are much more flexible than they were before your workout.

Static Stretches

Overhead Stretch (Shoulders and Arms)

Perform this stretch either standing or sitting in an upright position. Move one arm over your head and bend it, so your hand lies between your shoulder blades. Grasp your elbow with your other hand and gently pull your elbow toward your head until you feel a stretch in your shoulder and tricep. Try to keep your bicep as close to your ear as you can and hold the stretch for around 30 seconds, then repeat with your other arm.

The Cross-Body Stretch (Shoulders and Arms)

Stand upright and straighten your right arm out in front of you. Using your left forearm, gently pull your right arm in and across your chest. You will feel a significant stretch at the top and back of your right shoulder. Make sure your arm does not exceed your shoulder height. Hold the stretch for around 30 seconds then repeat this on the other side.

Reclined Back Stretch and Spinal Twist (Back)

Perform this stretch by lying flat on your back with your arms straight out to the side, so your body is in a T-shape. Keep your shoulders flat on the ground while you bring your right knee up to your chest, and then slowly lower it across your extended left leg. Make sure to keep your shoulders flat on the ground and don't worry if your right foot doesn't touch the ground. Hold this stretch for around 30 seconds before bringing your right leg back across your body and repeating this movement with your left leg.

Pectoral Stretch (Chest)

Stand upright and place your hands behind your buttocks with your palms facing away from your body and interlock your fingers. Bring your shoulder blades together and slowly lift your arms out behind you, while keeping them straight. Keep lifting your arms until you feel a stretch in your chest and hold this stretch for around 30 seconds. Alternatively, you can perform this stretch by holding on to each end of a rolled towel and extending your arms out behind your back.

The Bent-Over Hamstring Stretch (Legs)

Stand upright or sit on the floor with your feet together. Slowly bend forward and try to touch your toes with your fingertips (or get as close as you comfortably can). Hold this stretch for around 30 seconds.

Heel Drop Calf Stretches (Legs)

Stand upright on the edge of a raised surface such as a step. Shuffle your feet back until your heels are hanging off the edge and the balls of your feet are still on the surface. Lift your left foot and place it on your right heel to help keep your balance. Slowly lower your right foot down until you can feel a stretch in your right calf. You can hold on to a stable surface to keep you balanced if needed. Hold this stretch for around 30 seconds and then repeat it on the other side.

Standing Quad Stretch (Legs)

Stand up straight and place your feet about hip-width apart, lift your right leg off the ground and bend your right knee so your heel is close to your buttocks. Balance on your left leg, grasp your right foot with your right hand and gently pull it closer to your buttocks until you feel a stretch in your upper thigh. Hold this stretch for 30 seconds and then repeat on the other side. You can use a chair or a wall for support if you are worried about losing your balance.

The Straddle (Legs and Back)

Sit on the floor and extend your legs out in front of you in a wide V-shape. Lean forward slowly with your arms extended out in front of you and continue moving forward until you feel a significant stretch in your inner thighs and lower back. Hold this position for around 30 seconds and come up slowly when you are finished. As your flexibility increases, you will notice that you can reach further forward.

Downward-Facing Dog (Back and Legs)

For yoga lovers, this will be a very familiar stretch. Start in a high plank position, with your hands directly underneath your shoulders and extend your legs behind you, ensuring that they are about hip-width apart. Stabilize your core, contract your abdominal muscles (pull your belly button to your spine) and lift your buttocks toward the ceiling. Ensure that your feet and hands don't move during this process. Keep your back and legs straight and try to lower your heels down towards the ground as far as you can comfortably go. During this process, relax your neck and let your head hang down. Direct your gaze toward your feet and hold this for around 60 seconds.

KEY PRINCIPLES OF TRAINING

If you want to get the most out of your workouts, there are a few fundamental principles that every top trainer uses to design their workout routines. Regardless of whether you are an Olympic athlete or a home-exerciser, these universal principles are essential to help you achieve your health and fitness goals.

SPORRT

SPORRT stands for specificity, progression, overload, reversibility, rest, and tedium. They are the key elements required for a successful workout routine.

Specificity is important because, as obvious as this sounds, if you want to strengthen a particular set of muscles, you need to use exercises that target those muscles. For example, you need to perform exercises that target the arm muscles if you want to train your arms. This is where people who use bodyweight exercises thrive because most of the bodyweight exercises use multiple muscle groups, so individual exercises can target many areas at once.

Progression and **overload** are the second and third elements in SPORRT and are very closely linked together. Progressive overload is essential as you need to gradually increase the stress you're putting your body through to further your development. For example, weightlifters need to gradually increase the weight they are lifting; otherwise they will not get any stronger. You can progressively overload your body by altering three different aspects of your workouts: the frequency, intensity and duration.

- Frequency – this refers to the number of times throughout the week you are going to be exercising. For example,

increasing the frequency could mean going from exercising
three times a week to four times a week.

- Intensity – this refers to how hard you are working when you
  are exercising. For example, this could mean increasing the
  weight used in strength training, running at a pace where
  your heart rate is at 170 beats per minute instead of 150 beats
  per minute or adding in more exercises to a home workout
  routine.

- Duration – this refers to how long you spend doing a
  particular exercise. For example, this could mean swimming
  non-stop for 30 minutes instead of 20 minutes or performing
  home workout exercises for 60 seconds instead of 45
  seconds.

It is important to progressively overload your body gradually because
changing these elements too quickly can lead to injuries. Injuries can
take a long time to heal, and although the human body is an amaz-
ingly complex organism, some injuries can have lasting effects. When
you change the frequency, intensity or duration of your training,
make sure that you don't change all three at once. Instead, focus on
changing one of them and see how things go from there. Progressive
overload is a gradual process – don't rush it.

The fourth element is **reversibility**. Exercise is an ongoing lifestyle
choice, and it is not intended to have a cancellation date (unless you
are ill or injured when resting aids your recovery). If you exercise
consistently but then suddenly stop, your joint mobility, muscle
strength, and overall fitness will begin to decline. Regular exercise is
crucial to maintain your overall health and fitness.

One of the most important aspects of the SPORRT acronym is its fifth
element, which is the principle of **rest** and recovery. A common
problem that occurs is that people don't give themselves enough rest
in between their workouts, as they believe the more they do, the fitter
they will become. Overtraining can actually have an adverse effect on
your body and can cause more harm than good. Your body needs

time to recover from exercise to give those micro-tears that occur in the muscle enough time to heal, and for the muscle to rebuild itself stronger than it was before. However, this doesn't happen overnight. Generally, a day is enough time for most people to recover, but if you would like to exercise every day, then breaking up your routine can help prevent overtraining. For example, you could focus on upper body workouts on one day and lower body workouts the next.

The final element is **tedium,** aka boredom. A lack of variety in the way you exercise can quickly turn your routines into a repetitive rut. Adding a variety of different exercises and frequently mixing them up can help keep you motivated and ensure your exercise regime remains interesting. This doesn't mean completely revolutionizing your workout every single time but making slight changes to the type of exercise you are doing. For example, instead of doing standard push-ups every time you work out, mix it up by doing decline push-ups in one session, incline and diamond in another. Little changes like this can help prevent your workouts seeming like a chore or a punishment and can make them much more enjoyable.

HYDRATION

Water makes up around 60% of the human body and alongside oxygen, it is one of the most important nutrients for our bodies. When we exercise, the body loses water at a much quicker rate from a combination of sweating and an increased breathing rate. We also lose other nutrients and electrolytes when we exercise, and this can lead to dehydration.

Dehydration occurs when your body has less water than it needs and as a result, it can't function as efficiently as it usually would. When we are dehydrated, we quickly start to feel tired. Dehydration can affect your cognition and make you feel confused and irritable, as well as causing other symptoms such as headaches, a dry mouth and muscle cramps. An excellent measure of how hydrated you are is by observing the color of your urine. If it looks colorless or a very light yellow, then you are well hydrated. However, if it is a very dark yellow, that is a sign of dehydration.

Whether you are an Olympic athlete or someone who exercises to stay fit and healthy, hydration as a whole is vital, especially during exercise to prevent dehydration. There is no set amount of water you should drink each day as it can depend very much on different factors such as where you live and how hot it is, how much you sweat and also how much exercise you do and how intense it is. A rough guide to follow is taking your body weight (in pounds) and dividing that value by 2. This gives you a rough estimate of how much water you should be drinking (in ounces). For example, someone who is 160 pounds (72.5 kg) should be drinking around 80 ounces of water (around 2.3 liters of water) per day.

When exercising, the average person should be aiming for:

- Around 17-20 ounces (500 to 600 ml) of water two to three hours before an exercise session
- Around 8 ounces (230 to 250 ml) of water at the start of an exercise session
- Around 7 to 10 ounces (200 to 300 ml) of water every 10 to 20 minutes during the exercise session
- Around 8 ounces (230 to 250 ml) of water in the 30 minutes after you have finished exercising

For those who do intense exercise for a long period of time, an energy drink may be beneficial to help provide calories and replace some of the electrolytes lost during exercise such as potassium and sodium. Be careful what you drink and make sure to check the labels because some energy drinks have more sugar than others and depending on the recommended serving size, the values in the nutrition section may be more than you expect. However, for the majority of the time, water is all you need.

2

ARM EXERCISES

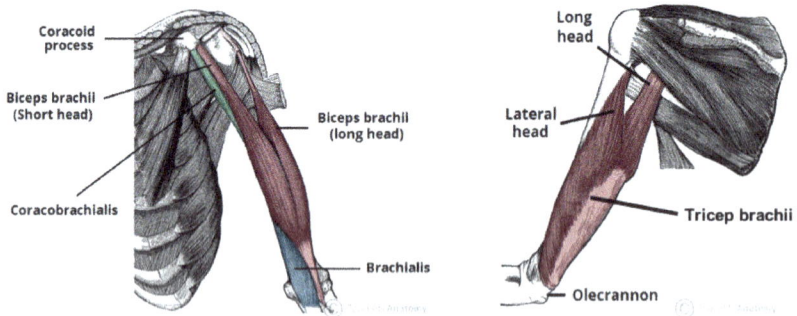

Photo of the biceps brachii (left) and the triceps brachii (right)

There are two main muscles in the upper arm that people target during their workouts: the biceps brachii and triceps brachii. The bicep muscle was named because it is a two-headed muscle and it is located at the front of the upper arm. These two heads start in the shoulder and then join together at the elbow, and its primary function is to bend the arm at the elbow joint.

The triceps are located at the back of the upper arm and acquired its name because the muscle has three heads. The primary function of the triceps is to straighten the arm at the elbow joint.

THE BENEFITS OF STRENGTHENING YOUR ARMS

Building the strength in your arms has more benefits than just the aesthetic appeal of having big strong arms. Arm exercises can have a conditioning effect on your cardiovascular system, and research has shown that bodyweight exercises which focus on muscle groups in the arms can strengthen the heart muscle and reduce your chances of developing heart disease.

There is a belief that strong legs are the only thing runners need to be successful. However, this isn't the case. Training your arms can help you run faster, improve your endurance and indirectly improve your posture. Working on your arms not only makes carrying heavy items easier, but it can also strengthen your bones and reduce the chances of developing osteoporosis (low bone density) later on in life.

———

PUSH-UPS

One of the most effective upper-body and core workouts that you can do are push-ups. This exercise incorporates multiple muscle groups and is a great way to build strength and get your heart rate up. Push-ups mainly target the pectoral muscles, but they also work the triceps, shoulder muscles and your core muscles.

The first thing you need to remember about push-ups is that there are no shortcuts. If you don't perform them correctly, sadly they're not going to have any effect. There are ways to increase or decrease the difficulty of these exercises, but the fundamentals will always remain the same.

There is no set number of push-ups that you should be aiming to do as everyone is different when it comes to strength. Instead, aim to do as many as you can with the proper technique, as you will benefit much more from doing fewer reps with proper technique than you would from doing double the number of push-ups but taking shortcuts.

Technique

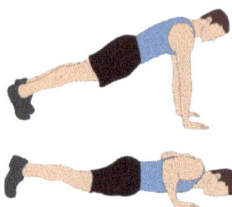

To perform a push-up, position your hands shoulder-width apart with your fingers facing forward, your arms straight and your feet together. Engage your core, slowly bend your arms and lower yourself down to the ground, exhaling as you go down and inhaling as you come up. Hold this position for a few seconds then push yourself back up to the starting position.

It is important to keep your body straight throughout the entire exercise. If you have your buttocks too high in the air or your pelvis hanging low towards the ground, you are not fully activating your core. Always ensure that you contract your abdominal muscles throughout this process by squeezing your belly button into your spine as this activates the majority of your core muscles.

Also, you need to make sure you are lowering your body far enough down towards the ground. Only slightly bending your arms isn't going to work the muscles in your chest or arms in their full range of motion. Commonly, the aim is to try and bend your arms so that your chest is only a few inches off the ground. However, in reality, everyone is different chest-wise, so a much more effective way to do push-ups is to lower yourself until there is a straight line from your elbow to your shoulder.

If you struggle to perform regular push-ups, start with some knee push-ups instead. This will help to build your strength and confidence. However, it is important to note that there is minimal core muscle activation with these types of push-ups. It will be more beneficial to perform regular push-ups from the beginning, and once you start struggling and feel tired, drop down to your knees and continue with knee push-ups. If you find your knees are hurting, put a pillow underneath them to make the exercise more comfortable.

There are several different types of push-up that you can do to make the exercise more varied and alter which muscles you are focusing on. The three main variations are the diamond push-up, incline push-up and decline push-up.

Diamond Push-Ups

The placement of your hands during your push-up routine will determine which muscles are predominantly used during the exercise. Standard push-ups work the triceps, shoulders, and chest relatively equally, but if you want to attempt a push-up that will help to build your triceps more, the diamond push-up is a great exercise to try.

This exercise is more advanced than regular push-ups and may take a while to accomplish if you are just starting. Diamond push-ups get their name from the diamond shape your hands make when they come together.

To perform a diamond push-up, start in the standard push-up position and then move your hands together until your index fingers are touching while pointing forward and your thumbs are touching while pointing backwards. You will notice that this hand placement produces a diamond-shaped gap between your hands. Engage your core and bend your arms to lower yourself down towards the ground. Hold this position for a few seconds and then push yourself back up to the starting position.

This push-up position may make you feel unsteady. If this is the case, you can position your feet slightly wider as this will help you maintain your balance.

Incline and Decline Push-Ups

Incline and decline push-ups work by increasing the height of your feet or your hands. Incline push-ups will require you to put your hands on something higher than the floor such as a stable chair or bed and continue with your basic push-up technique.

Decline push-ups are significantly more difficult than incline push-ups and require a greater level of strength. Decline push-ups involve raising your feet to a level higher than your body, which increases the difficulty of the push-up.

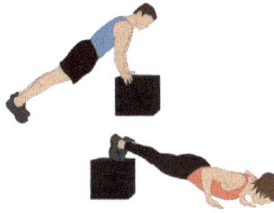

Both incline and decline push-ups work your shoulders, chest, and triceps but in slightly different ways. Incline push-ups predominantly target the lower chest and back muscles due to the angle of your body during the exercise. On the other hand, decline push-ups primarily target the upper chest muscles and deltoids. Compared to regular push-ups, where you are lifting around 70% of your body weight, you are pushing more of your body weight with the decline push-up; the higher your feet are, the more of your body weight you are pushing.

CRAB WALK

The crab walk is a very unusual exercise, and even though it seems like it is part of a game that kids would play, it is an excellent workout for the triceps. It also works the shoulders, chest, core, glutes, hamstrings and quads.

Even though you might not be moving very quickly, you will feel your heart rate increase, making this exercise a surprisingly good one to add to your cardio routine. Don't be disheartened if you can't hold the position for very long in the beginning stages; it will become easier as your strength and fitness levels improve.

Another added benefit of the crab walk is that it stretches your pectoral muscles. This helps to activate the muscle fibers in the chest and may help to relieve any underlying stiffness from previous exercises.

Technique

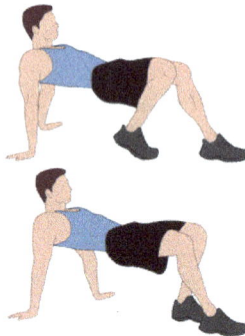

To perform this exercise, start by sitting on the floor with your hands flat behind you. Ensure that your fingertips are facing out to the side, bend your knees and plant the soles of your feet firmly on the ground. Lift your hips off the ground to raise your body into the crab position and distribute your body weight equally between your arms and legs. Then walk up and down in this position. The higher you elevate your hips, the more you will activate your core and the harder the movement will be.

———

TRICEP DIPS

Tricep dips are so named because they are an extremely effective exercise for working the triceps on the back of your arms. They also target the trapezius, pectoralis major and serratus anterior.

As with most exercises, you must ensure that you have thoroughly warmed up and stretched before attempting tricep dips, because this is an exercise that can result in injury if it is not performed correctly or without adequate preparation. I suggest you perform this exercise closer to the end of your workout routine because your muscles will be sufficiently warmed up by then.

Technique

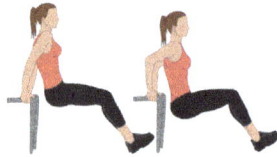

To perform tricep dips, you will need a bed, stable chair or any other flat surface. Sit down on the edge of the stable surface and place your hands shoulder-width apart with your fingertips pointing out behind you. Positioning your hands with your fingers facing forward or placing your hands wider than shoulder-width will significantly increase strain on other joints, especially the shoulder joint. Engage your core, bend your arms and slowly dip down until your arms are at a 90-degree angle. Make sure to keep your elbows in and don't let them stray out to the side. Once you have dipped down, hold this position for a couple of seconds and then push yourself back up to the starting position. Make sure to keep a slight bend in your arms and don't lock them at the top of the movement because locking your arms will prevent your triceps from working throughout the whole exercise.

There are several variations of the tricep dip, and you can choose which one you do according to your current strength level. The difficulty of each variation depends on the positioning of your legs. However, the technique stays the same regardless of which one you choose to do.

Beginner (tricep dip with knees bent) – This is the exercise shown in the diagram above. Place your hands flat behind you, put your feet together flat on the floor and bend your knees. Slowly dip down until your arms are at 90-degrees and then push yourself back up to the starting position.

Intermediate (tricep dip with legs straight) - Place your hands flat behind you, extend your legs out in front of you and rest your weight on your heels. Slowly dip down until your arms are at 90-degrees and then push yourself back up to the starting position.

Advanced (tricep dip with legs raised) – Place your hands flat behind you and place your legs on a surface which is at the same height as your hands and bend your knees slightly. Slowly dip down until your arms are at 90-degrees and then push yourself back up to the starting position.

Expert (tricep dip using parallel bars) – Place your hands on two bars (or any other suitable surface such as the backs of two chairs) and raise your body off the ground until your arms are straight. Keep your chest and chin up, cross your feet behind you and slowly dip down until your arms are bent at 90-degrees before pushing yourself back up to the starting position. If you want to make this exercise even more challenging, you can add weights to your feet, such as a bag with some books in it and perform the exercise that way.

You may feel a burning sensation in your triceps practically from the first or second dip but don't let this stop you. Remember that the body is more resilient than people think. If you keep including this exercise into your routine, you will quickly see why it is one of the best exercises for building your triceps.

TRICEP EXTENSIONS

Similar to the diamond push-up and tricep dips, this exercise is great for targeting your triceps. It may look like an easy exercise, but don't be fooled, it is much harder than it seems. Don't let that stop you though. The more you practice it, the better you will get.

Technique

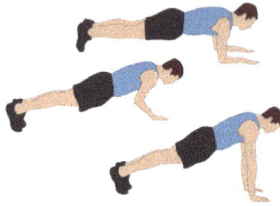

To perform tricep extensions, get into a plank position (the top image above) with your forearms flat on the ground in front of you, your feet straight out behind you and your back straight. Make sure to keep your core engaged and don't let your hips sag down. From here, push down into the ground to raise your body until your arms are fully extended. Hold this position for a few seconds then slowly lower yourself down into the plank position again.

If you are struggling to push your body weight up, try performing this exercise on your knees instead. This is a great way to get yourself accustomed to the movement and build up the strength required to complete the full movement.

———

BICEP CURLS

If you want to focus on your biceps and would like to add some extra tone and muscle mass, a great exercise is the bicep curl. If you already have dumbbells at home then you can use these, but if you don't, filled water bottles work just as well. Don't use unopened carbonated drinks for this exercise... that is a disaster waiting to happen!

Technique

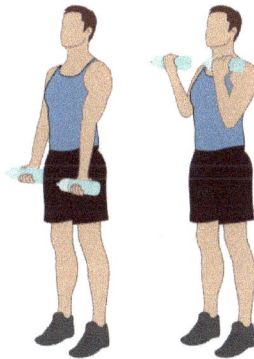

To perform a bicep curl, hold the weights in each hand and rest your arms by your side. Keep your elbows close to your body and have your palms facing upward. Slowly raise the weights towards your shoulder without moving your upper arm and exhale as you do so. Hold this position for a couple of seconds at the top of the movement and then slowly lower the weight back down until your arm is straight again, inhaling as you do so.

The weight used for this exercise can be increased as your strength improves. If the water bottles you are using become too easy, you can gradually increase the weight by using larger water bottles, bags of flour, heavy books or other household items.

UNDERHAND CHIN-UP/UNDERHAND INVERTED ROW

Chin-ups and pull-ups are renowned for being two of the best exercises for training your arms, shoulders and back muscles, and they are two exercises that people tend to either love or hate. A lot of people can struggle to complete a single rep, whilst others can keep going until the cows come home. The most important thing to remember is that the only way to get better at them is to practice. They are also great exercises to do to measure the progress of your strength training. It is incredibly satisfying to see the number of repetitions you can perform increase over time.

Despite being two very similar looking exercises, they do have their differences. One of the key differences between the exercises is the type of grip you use. When performing a chin-up, you use an underhand grip (where your palms are facing towards you) with your hands about shoulder-width apart, whereas when performing a pull-up, you use an overhand grip (where your palms face away from you) with your hands slightly wider than shoulder-width. While both exercises will work your arms, shoulders and back, the difference in grip means that you work certain muscles more than others. Chin-ups will focus more on training your biceps, whereas pull-ups will focus more on training your latissimus dorsi in your back. Other additional benefits of these exercises are that they can improve your grip strength and they can help improve your posture, making it beneficial for those who have a problem with slouching. We are going to focus on chin-ups now, and pull-ups will be discussed later on in Chapter 5.

A pull-up bar isn't essential to perform these exercises, but it is a great investment. Make sure to check that it is properly secured to the wall or door frame before you use it. However, as you'll have read from the title of this book, you don't need equipment to perform these movements, and I will also show you a method to train the same muscles without using a pull-up bar.

Underhand Chin-up

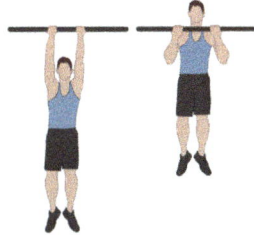

To perform a chin-up, reach your arms up and grasp the bar (or other surface) with your hands shoulder-width apart and your palms facing towards you. Slightly squeeze your shoulder blades together, bend your arms and pull yourself up until your chin has passed the bar. Have your legs positioned slightly in front of your body, point your toes towards the ground with your knees nice and straight. This leg positioning will help ensure your body is streamlined. Make sure to keep your back straight, your chest up and engage your core as this will help make you more stable and less likely to swing. Once you are at the top of the motion, hold it for a few seconds before slowly lowering yourself back down to your starting position. Inhale as you lift yourself up to the bar and then exhale as you lower yourself back down.

Underhand Inverted Row

If there is a park nearby with some raised bars or some low tree branches, you can use those and apply the same technique as I have described above. Just make sure they are sturdy enough to support your weight. However, if you don't have anything like that nearby, a great way to work the same muscles without using a bar is to do an underhand inverted row.

To perform this exercise, you need a sturdy table (one that isn't going to break or flip over if you apply weight to it) or a low railing. Position yourself under the table or railing with your chest directly underneath, grasp it with your hands shoulder-width apart using an under-hand grip and straighten your legs so you are resting on your heels. Keep your whole body straight, engage your core and then pull your-self up to the table/bar as high as you can whilst keeping your heels on the ground. Hold this position for a few seconds before lowering yourself back down to the starting position. If you are using a table, make sure you don't bump your head. To make this exercise easier, place your feet flat on the ground and perform the movement that way. Alternatively, you can make this exercise harder by raising your feet onto a chair and performing the inverted row that way.

———

3

SHOULDER EXERCISES

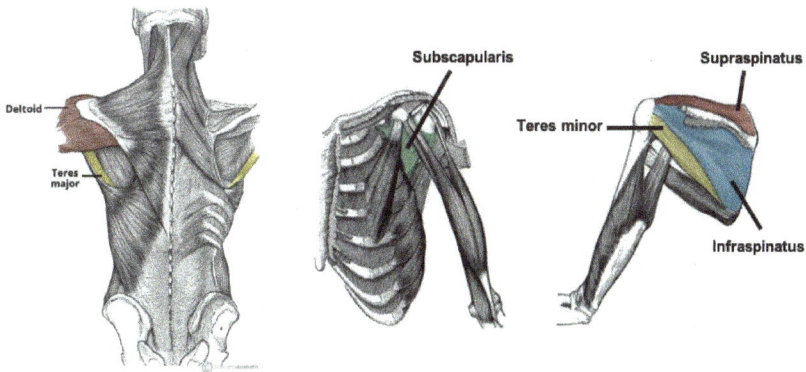

Photo of the deltoid (left) and the rotator cuff muscles (middle and right)

Along with your triceps, your deltoids are involved in many upper body exercises. Your deltoid is that nice large muscle at the top of your arm and shoulder, and it is the muscle commonly used for injections. It was given its name because of its shape resembling the Greek letter for delta (Δ). The deltoid can be divided into anterior, middle and posterior regions, and its primary function is to lift the arm forwards, backwards and outwards.

The other shoulder muscles discussed in this chapter are the rotator cuff muscles. The rotator cuff is made up of four individual muscles: the supraspinatus, infraspinatus, subscapularis and teres minor. These muscles help to stabilise the shoulder joint, rotate the arm and minorly assist the deltoid with lifting your arm outwards. There are other muscles that make up the extrinsic muscles in the shoulder such as the trapezius, but they will be covered in Chapter 5 as most of these muscles are targeted during back exercises. The shoulder exercises included in this section will focus on the deltoids and the rotator cuff muscles.

THE BENEFITS OF STRENGTHENING YOUR SHOULDERS

Working on your shoulders can help give you a more muscular frame, but there are more benefits to having strong shoulder than just how they look. Strong shoulders allow you to move your arms with greater ease, increase the amount of strength that you can naturally put into physical tasks, and you will be able to carry much heavier everyday items with greater ease. By strengthening your shoulders, you will be able to increase the speed at which your arms can move too. Strong shoulders make everyday tasks easier like when your spouse calls you to assist with carrying in the groceries from the car, when you're throwing a ball for your dog or when you're hitting a "birdie" on the golf course (1 under par, not the flying animal).

The shoulder joint has an extensive range of motion due to it being a ball and socket joint. As a result, it is one of the weakest joints in the body. If the muscles surrounding it are weak, the normal range of motion can be adversely affected, resulting in injury. Keeping these muscles healthy can help prevent this from happening.

———

SHADOWBOXING

At first glance, it might seem strange that shadowboxing is in here, but it can have a significant effect on your shoulder development as well as your overall fitness. It also works the muscles in your arms, chest, core and legs and shadowboxing doubles up as a fantastic cardio exercise, causing the heart rate to shoot up and helping to burn unwanted fat. You can also include shadowboxing as part of your warm-up routine. Even if you never plan on setting foot in a boxing ring, it is a great exercise to help improve your overall fitness. It is also an enjoyable exercise, especially if you are a fan of Muhammad Ali or the movies "Rocky" and "Real Steel."

If you happen to have a punching bag, it is perfect for this exercise. However, if you don't have one, don't worry as you can use the same technique while boxing the air. Just make sure there aren't any breakable or fragile objects nearby likes vases and lamps.

Technique

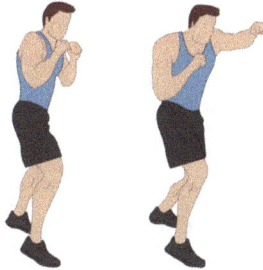

To start, you will need to adopt a boxing stance and there are two types you can choose: the traditional stance and the southpaw stance. To get into the **traditional stance**, position your right foot slightly behind you and place your left foot forward (so your feet are diagonal from each other), have your feet shoulder-width apart, bend your knees and slightly rotate your torso to the right, so your left side is out in front. Raise your hands to your chin, slightly dip your chin, keep your elbows pointing down and slightly raise your shoulders (but not too high that they are shrugged up to your ears).

If this stance doesn't feel comfortable, you can use **the southpaw stance** which is illustrated in the diagram above. To get into this stance, you reverse the traditional stance by positioning your right foot forward and your left foot behind your body, and rotating your body to the left, so your right side is out in front. Again, raise your hands to your chin, slightly dip your chin, keep your elbows pointing down and slightly raise your shoulders.

There are several different types of punch you can do in boxing. For the purpose of these exercises, I am going to describe the punches in the traditional stance as this is the stance that is most commonly used. To perform these punches in the southpaw stance, reverse the movements and punch with the opposite hand to the one I am describing below.

The first type of punch is the **jab** which is the quickest and most common punch in boxing, and it generates the majority of its power from the deltoid. A jab is a straight punch with the lead hand positioned out in front of your body. When you are in the traditional stance, punching with your left hand would be your jab and vice versa for the southpaw stance. When you jab, fully extend your arm out in front of your body and slightly rotate your hips to the right. Make sure to keep your elbow straight and don't let it stray out to the side. Once you have fully extended your arm, snap it back into your body.

The second type of punch is the **cross** which is the most powerful punch you can do. A cross is a punch with the rear hand that travels across your body; hence the name. When performing a cross, fully extend your right arm out in front of you and simultaneously rotate your body to the left while pivoting on your right foot, so your heel is off the ground (as if you are stubbing out a cigarette). This rotation of the body helps to provide your punch with more power.

The third type of punch you can do is the **uppercut**. An uppercut is a power punch in which you punch your arm in an upward motion. When performing an uppercut, you need to use the correct hand positioning. Hold your right arm out in front of you with your palm facing up, bend your elbow until it is at 90-degrees and make a fist. To perform a right uppercut, adopt this hand position and punch upwards while twisting your body to the left and pivoting on your right foot. To perform a left uppercut, perform the same movement but rotate your body to the right while pivoting on your left foot. The power in this punch comes from a combination of twisting your hips, snapping your shoulder into the punch and tightening your core muscles.

The last type of punch is the **hook**. A hook is where you punch in a horizontal arc shape from the side. When performing a hook, you need to use the correct hand positioning. Hold your right arm out to the side, bend your elbow until it is at a 90-degree angle and make a fist with your thumb on top. To perform a right hook, adopt this hand position and punch by rotating your hips to the left while pivoting on your right foot. To perform a left hook, repeat the same movement but twist your body to the right while pivoting on your left foot. A lot of people think the correct way to perform the hook is to stand still and swing your arm in an arc. However, the proper way to perform the hook is to keep your arm stationary and rotate your torso and hips to deliver the punch. The rotation of your body generates the force that gives your punch its power.

If you want to focus more on speed, then you can perform combinations with mainly crosses and jabs, but if you would prefer to focus more on power, use combinations that include uppercuts and hooks. Alternatively, you can do a mixture of the four. Here are some very basic combinations you can use as part of your workout. Again, these are in the traditional stance so reverse the movements if you want to use the southpaw stance.

1. Left jab – right cross
2. Right cross – left jab
3. Left jab – left jab – right cross
4. Left jab – right cross – left jab
5. Left jab – right cross – left hook
6. Left jab – right cross – left hook – right cross
7. Right cross – left hook – right uppercut
8. Left jab – right uppercut – left hook

If you want to make this exercise even more challenging, you can grab some light dumbbells (if you have them) or filled water bottles and hold these while you punch. Since you don't have an opponent firing punches back at you, you can focus more on your form and power to help develop your shoulders.

———

SHOULDER EXERCISES | 47

SHOULDER PRESS

This exercise is one of the best for building your deltoids (notably the anterior region) as well as focusing on your triceps, trapezius and your pectoralis muscles. The movement of this exercise also indirectly works your core muscles, which are activated to help keep your body straight and balanced. The shoulder press can be performed using dumbbells (if you have them) but filled water bottles, bags of flour and other household items are equally as effective for this exercise.

When choosing a weight (whether it's a dumbbell or household item), make sure to start light, almost as if you feel like it is too light. This is because the shoulder press can be challenging once you reach the middle of a set and using a weight that is too heavy could injure your shoulders if you get tired and stop focusing on using the proper technique.

Technique

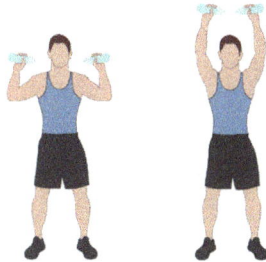

You can perform this exercise either sitting or standing, but it is easier to maintain your posture when in a seated position. Stand/sit up straight and hold a weight in each hand at shoulder height, with your palms facing forwards. Position your arms so they are in a 90-degree angle at your elbows, making your upper body into a U-shape. Keep your back straight, your chest up and your core engaged. Slowly straighten your arms above your head, hold for a few seconds at the top of the movement and then slowly bring your arms back down to the U-shaped position. To get the most contraction out of your shoulder muscles, do not fully straighten your arms or touch the weights together. Also, keep your wrists in line with your forearms and don't let your elbows creep forward. You want to have a straight line going across both your shoulders.

This exercise might feel challenging at first because your shoulders won't get a break. In contrast to a shoulder press machine at the gym, where your arms are in a rested position from the start and the muscles are only engaged when you straighten your arms, this exercise will keep your muscles activated throughout the whole movement.

———

HANDSTAND PUSH-UP

As intimidating and challenging as handstand push-ups sound, don't skip this page and move on to the next one because this is a beneficial exercise. It helps to build up strength in your deltoids, pectoral muscles and your trapezius and targets your core and glutes too. This exercise is significantly more challenging than previous exercises, mainly because it requires a lot of core activation and strength needed to complete it; however, you are entirely capable of doing it. All you need to do is build up to it.

Ideally, this type of exercise should be interspersed throughout your workout routines because, unlike flying mammals such as bats, human beings are not designed to spend too much time upside down. Being in an inverted position for too long can cause headaches and dizziness from the blood rush to the head. If you do start to experience these types of symptoms, it is better to stop the exercise and wait for the symptoms to clear. However, since we are going to be slowly building up to a full handstand push-up, this will help you get used to the feeling of being upside down.

Warm-up

Before you begin, you need to warm up your wrists. Having the wrists cocked back isn't a normal day-to-day position for most people, so it is important to properly warm them up to avoid any discomfort when holding your body weight up. I would recommend you do these exercises before you start:

Wrist extension and flexion stretch – Straighten your right arm out in front of you and cock your wrist back, so your fingers are pointing up to the ceiling. Grasp onto your fingers with your left hand and pull your hand back until you feel a stretch in your wrist and the underside of your forearm. Hold this stretch for 30 seconds. Release the stretch and bend your wrist down so your fingers are pointing towards the floor and your palm is facing towards you. Grasp your fingers and pull them toward you, until you feel a stretch in your wrist and the top of your forearm. Hold for 30 seconds and then repeat on the other side.

Kneeling floor wrist extension – Get down on all fours with your hands and knees evenly spaced, your palms flat on the floor in front of you and your fingers spread apart facing forwards. Make sure to fully straighten your arm so your elbows are locked and slowly lean your body forward as far as you can go without hurting your wrists or taking your palms off the floor. Either hold this position or rock back and forth for 15 seconds. Next, go back to the original position and rotate your hands so they are facing towards you. This time move your body back as far as you can go without hurting your wrists or taking your palms off the floor. Again, do this for 15 seconds and either hold the position or rock back and forth.

Figure of 8 – Clasp your hands together with your right thumb on top and bring your elbows in so your forearms are against each other in front of you. Keep your arms still and move your wrists in a figure of 8 motion for 30 seconds. Do not be alarmed if you hear any cracking or popping noises. Unclasp your fingers then clasp your hands together again with your left thumb on top and perform this movement for 30 seconds.

Now you have warmed up your wrists, you are ready for the hand-stand push-up.

Technique

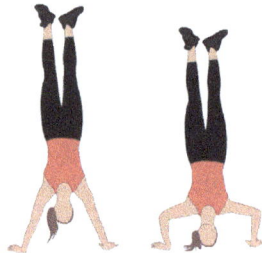

The best way to build up to a full handstand push-up is to follow the route of exercises below, as these will help you build the upper body strength required. You can start at the step you feel is appropriate for you and you can build up this exercise as far as you want. When performing any of these exercises, it is beneficial to have a pillow or other soft item underneath your head because this can help prevent any injuries if you lose control of your descent and fall.

Beginner (Pike Push-up) – This exercise is great for those wanting to build up their upper body strength and their confidence to move on to the next step. To perform the pike push-up, start by getting into the downward dog position, where your hands are shoulder-width apart, your head is dropped down between your arms, your legs are extended behind you (resting your weight on the tip of your toes) and your buttocks are raised into the air. If done correctly, your body should look like it is in an A-shape. Contract your abdominal muscles, keep your shoulders pulled back and slowly bend your elbows, bringing yourself down towards the ground. Go as low as you comfortably can, but you want to aim to bend your elbows until they are at a 90-degree angle. Hold this position for a few seconds then push yourself back up to your original position.

Intermediate (Elevated Pike Push-up) – Get into the downward dog position but this time, place your feet on a raised surface such as a chair, step or box. Contract your abdominal muscles, keep your shoulders pushed back and bend your elbows. Slowly lower yourself down to the ground and aim for that 90-degree angle at your elbow. Hold this position for a few seconds then push yourself back up to your original position.

Advanced (Wall Handstand Push-ups) – Stand with your back facing the wall and get into a traditional push-up position. Instead of having your feet resting on the ground, place them on the wall and walk them up to increase your height. The higher you go, the more difficult the push-up will be. I would recommend starting low at first and then gradually building up. Once you have chosen your desired height, bend your elbows and slowly lower yourself down to the ground. Make sure to contract your abdominal muscles, keep your shoulders back and aim for that 90-degree angle in your elbows. Hold this position for a few seconds and then push yourself back up to the original position. Once you are confident with walking yourself up the wall, repeat this exercise but invert your body position. Get into a handstand position with your heels resting against the wall and repeat the exercise this way.

Expert (Handstand Push-ups) – Once you are confident with the previous steps, it is time to do a full handstand push-up without a wall. Get into a handstand position and engage your core to help keep you balanced. Keep your shoulders back and bend your arms, slowly lowering yourself down to the ground. Hold this position for a few seconds then carefully push yourself back up to your original position. I would recommend having someone with you to help catch you if you start to fall over.

Being able to do a full handstand push-up without any support can take a long time to achieve; I am nowhere near being able to do a full handstand push-up. Don't put pressure on yourself to progress through all these stages. If you only want to progress as far as the elevated pike push-up then that is absolutely fine. Regardless of which exercise you choose, it will have a significant effect on your upper body strength.

———

SHOULDER EXERCISES | 53

DELTOID FLIES

A great exercise that you can use to target your deltoids is deltoid flies. This exercise also works your pectoral muscles, rotator cuff muscles and trapezius. Contrary to popular belief, you don't need to use heavy weights for noticeable results, especially when it comes to the deltoid fly.

Using a heavier weight increases the risk of injury as well as increasing the likelihood that you will need to "cheat" your way to completing the exercise. An example of this would be lifting your arm to a certain point and then leaning your body to the side or shrugging the shoulder to help raise the weight higher. These cheats help to raise the weight up higher, but the movement is assisted by other muscles and it is not achieved by the deltoids. It is much more beneficial to use a lighter weight and perform the technique correctly to work the deltoids fully. You can use light dumbbells, or household items like water bottles are also effective.

There are two variations of the deltoid fly: the lateral deltoid fly and the rear deltoid fly. Each of these exercises targets the deltoids, but they focus on different parts of the muscle. The lateral deltoid fly focusses more on the middle region of the deltoid, whereas the rear deltoid fly focusses more on the posterior region of the deltoid. Both are extremely effective exercises so we will be discussing both of them.

Technique

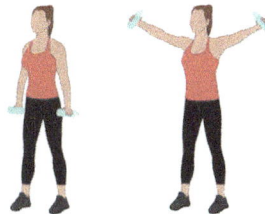

To perform the **lateral deltoid fly**, stand with your legs hip-width apart and have your arms at your sides with weights in each hand. Keep your back straight, engage your core and then slowly lift your arms out to the side. Make sure to slightly bend your arms and lift them until your hands are just above shoulder height. A common mistake is only raising your arms until they are at shoulder height. However, this doesn't fully contract the deltoid muscle, so try to lift your arms slightly higher than shoulder height. Once you have raised your arms beyond your shoulders, hold that position for a few seconds before slowly lowering your arms. Don't lower your arms down to your sides. Instead, lower them to around 30 to 45-degrees before repeating the movement as this will help ensure your deltoids work throughout the whole exercise. This is because the supraspinatus performs the first 15 degrees of this arc movement and then the deltoid takes over after that.

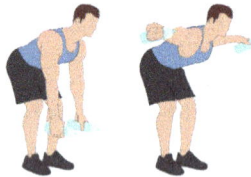

To perform the **rear deltoid fly**, stand with your legs hip-width apart, slightly bend your body forward at your hips, bend your knees and have your arms hanging down below your chest. Make sure to engage your core and keep your back straight; even though you are bent over, don't let your back arch. Slightly bend your arms and slowly raise them out to the side until your hands are above shoulder height. Hold this position for a few seconds before slowly lowering your arms back down. Again, lower your arms to around 30 to 45-degrees to help work your deltoid throughout the whole exercise.

———

ROTATOR CUFF STRENGTHENING EXERCISES

These stabilizing muscles are regularly unappreciated and typically go unnoticed; people are often unaware of their importance until they are injured. These small muscles may seem insignificant, but they play an integral role in the overall health and flexibility of the shoulder joint. A rotator cuff injury is one of the most common shoulder injuries that can occur as people get older, and if you think it takes significant force to damage these muscles, you would be mistaken.

Fortunately, the risk of these injuries occurring can be reduced by specifically exercising and strengthening the rotator cuff muscles. Unlike other exercises where you will gradually increase the weight over time, the weights used for the rotator cuff exercises need to remain relatively light, regardless of how strong and fit you become. In fact, these exercises can damage your rotator cuff muscles if you increase the weight beyond 2 or 3 pounds. Stick to a filled water bottle, a can of vegetables or a very light dumbbell.

We are going to be discussing two exercises which target the rotator cuff muscles: the full bow and the internal/external rotation.

Technique

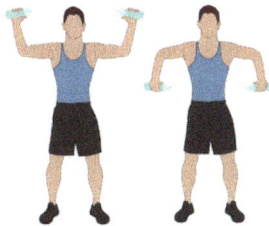

To perform the **full bow**, either stand or sit with a light weight in each hand. Raise your arms to shoulder height and bend your elbows to 90-degrees, making your upper body into a U-shape (similar to the starting position of the shoulder press). Make sure to keep your back straight, your core engaged and rotate your hands so that your palms are facing forwards. Slowly rotate your arms down until your hands are pointing downwards, making your body into an inverted U-shape. Hold this position for a few seconds then rotate your arms back to the original position.

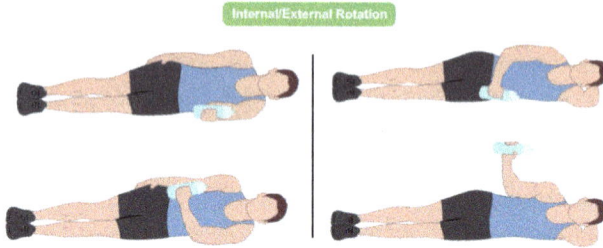

To perform the **internal/external rotation,** lie on one of your sides and support your head with your arm or a pillow. The side you work will depend on which side you are lying on. When you are lying on your right side, you will be performing external rotation of your left rotator cuff and internal rotation of your right rotator cuff. When you are lying on your left side, you will be performing external rotation of your right rotator cuff and internal rotation of your left rotator cuff. This might sound confusing, so I will use the left side as an example.

Lie on your left side and support your head with your left arm. Hold a light weight in your right hand, keep your right elbow bent at a 90-degree angle and tuck it in closely to your side. Slowly rotate your right forearm out from your body as far as you comfortably can and then slowly rotate it back in towards your body. This movement is external rotation of the right rotator cuff. Now switch the weight from your right hand to your left hand. Keep your elbow bent at 90-degrees and tucked in close to your side. Slowly rotate your left forearm in towards your body and then slowly rotate it back to the original position. This movement is internal rotation of the left rotator cuff. Repeat these exercises lying on your right side.

Incorporating these exercises into your routine once or twice a week will greatly increase the strength of your rotator cuff muscles. Although you may not see visible results, you will significantly reduce the chances of any future shoulder injuries occurring. Don't forget these little guys. Your future self will be very grateful!

———

4

CHEST EXERCISES

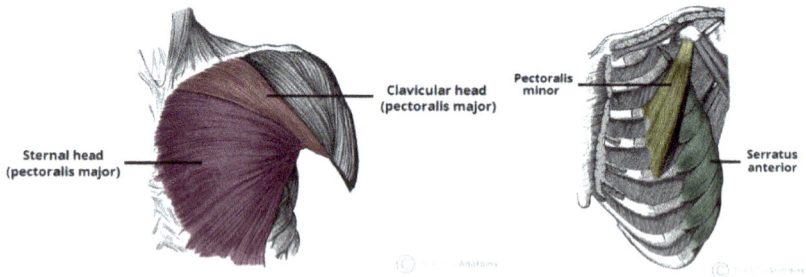

Photo of pectoralis major (left), pectoralis minor (right) and serratus anterior (right)

The main muscles in your chest are the pectoralis major, pectoralis minor and the serratus anterior. The pectoralis major is the large, superficial muscle which is very prominent on the chests of bodybuilders. It is responsible for bringing your arm in closer to your body and rotating your arm inwards. The pectoralis minor lies underneath the pectoralis major, and it is responsible for the forward movement and stabilization of the shoulder blades. Finally, your serratus anterior is located more on the side of your chest along your ribs. It is responsible for keeping the shoulder blades in place against the ribcage, as well as rotating the shoulder

CHEST EXERCISES | 59

blades as you lift your arm, allowing your arm to be raised above your head.

THE BENEFITS OF STRENGTHENING YOUR CHEST

As well as the aesthetic benefits of having a muscular chest, there are many other benefits to training these muscles. The chest houses some of the largest muscles in the body, and these muscles are used frequently in many upper body movements. Simple tasks like washing your hair, getting dressed and pulling open a door all involve the use of the chest muscles, so making sure they are strong will help make everyday tasks much easier.

As well as improving your overall upper body strength, the pectoralis muscles work with your back muscles to help give you good posture. Individuals who perform lots of free-weight chest exercises like the bench press can have issues with their posture. This is because they are over-exercising their chest, which can cause the pectoralis muscle to tighten, causing the shoulders to hunch forward. However, body-weight chest exercises don't have this effect because these exercises target many muscles in the upper body, particularly the shoulder, chest and upper back muscles. Individuals who stick to bodyweight exercises have less chance of developing any problems with their posture. If you want to keep your pectoralis muscles stretched, the pectoral stretch discussed in Chapter 1 is an effective method for doing so.

———

WIDE PUSH-UPS

This exercise is very similar to the traditional push-up already discussed in this book. However, this version of the push-up is much more challenging because of the wider positioning of the hands. By widening the distance between your hands, you are targeting the chest and shoulder muscles more than the traditional push-up does. The wider your hands are, the more your chest muscles have to work. As well as targeting your chest, shoulders and triceps, the wide push-up also targets your serratus anterior much more than a regular push-up. Not only does changing the width of your hand positioning add variety to your workouts, it also allows the muscles to go through a different range of motion and help reduce the risk of overuse injuries.

Technique

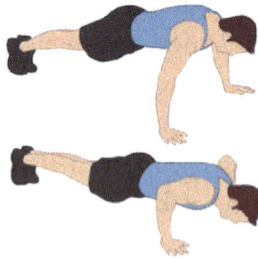

To perform the wide push-up, start in a standard push-up position where your hands are shoulder-width apart, your fingers are facing forward and your feet are together. Move your hands to the side, increasing the distance between them, engage your core, and slowly bend your arms to lower yourself down to the ground. Hold this position for a few seconds then push yourself back up to your original position.

Make sure to keep your back straight, don't let your pelvis sag or raise your buttocks into the air, and try to lower yourself down until your elbows are bent at 90-degrees and your arms are in line with your shoulders. Slightly bending your arms will not fully activate the chest muscles. As your chest muscles get stronger, gradually increase the distance between your hands to make the exercise more challenging.

If you need to, you can perform this exercise from your knees to help develop your strength. Alternatively, start with standard wide push-ups and then drop down to your knees once you begin to feel tired.

———

CLAP PUSH-UP

The clap push-up is an advanced exercise that involves propelling yourself into the air after each push-up, and targets the pectoralis muscles, triceps, shoulders and core muscles. The explosive nature of launching your body off the ground not only helps to burn fat and improve your cardiovascular fitness, it also activates the fast-twitch muscle fibers in your chest, shoulders and arms. Targeting these muscle fibers helps to maximize the effect of the workout on your muscles and increase the amount of muscle mass you develop.

Being able to launch yourself off the ground, clap your hands in mid-air, and return to a standard push-up position before falling face-first onto the floor might seem unlikely. However, the more you practice, the quicker your strength and confidence will increase, and this exercise will be easier and less scary. If you want to be safe, pop a pillow underneath your face to keep it looking pretty.

Technique

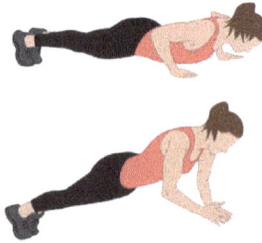

To perform this exercise, get into a push-up position with your hands shoulder-width apart, fingers facing forwards, back straight and feet together. Engage your core and slowly lower yourself down to the ground until your elbows are in line with your shoulders (like you would with a regular push-up). From here, push as explosively as possible to launch your upper body into the air and clap before (carefully) landing. Never land with your arms straight; you need to land softly with your arms slightly bent, ready to go straight into the next rep. Make sure you keep your back straight and push using your upper body only; don't let the momentum come from your hips.

If you want to build up the confidence and upper body strength required to do a full clap push-up, then you can make it easier in a few different ways. Start by performing a push-up from your knees without clapping, focusing on launching yourself into the air and landing softly. When doing this exercise on your knees, make sure you are leaning forward and using your upper body to perform the movement; it is very easy to rely on your hips to help lift your body up and down, which doesn't work the upper body. From there you can add in a clap when you feel more confident. Once you have perfected that, try a regular push-up but focus on launching yourself into the air and landing softly without clapping.

Explosive exercises like these are extremely effective at building muscle mass, but you can injure yourself if you don't have the upper body strength required or you perform them too often. Make sure to give yourself a few days to rest before doing these explosive push-ups again.

———

SPIDERMAN PUSH-UPS

Sadly, no matter how many of these push-ups you attempt, it won't turn you into your friendly neighborhood Spiderman. However, it is an effective exercise that targets your pectoral muscles, triceps and shoulders, while requiring you to focus on your core muscles as you control your descent. Spiderman push-ups require extreme muscle control and strength. They also help to develop your balance and core strength and take them to the next level.

Technique

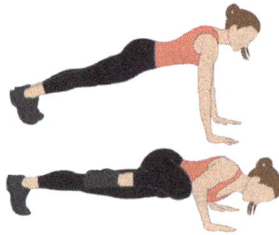

To perform this exercise, get into a standard push-up position by placing your hands slightly wider than shoulder-width apart, keeping your back straight and your feet together. Engage your core and bend your elbows to start slowly lowering yourself down towards the floor as if you were performing a standard push-up. As you start descending, lift your right foot off the ground and bring your right knee up towards your right elbow. You want to time this movement so that your knee reaches your elbow as you reach your lowest point and you are balancing using one foot. If you are doing it correctly, you should look like you are the masked superhero walking on a wall. Hold this position for a few seconds before pushing yourself back up to your original position while simultaneously placing your right leg back onto the ground. Repeat this movement by lifting your other leg.

If you want to make this exercise slightly easier, start by splitting the movement into different segments. Perform a regular push-up and once you have lowered yourself down to the ground, hold that position at the bottom and then bring your knee up to your elbow.

Alternatively, if you want to challenge yourself, try walking Spiderman push-ups. Start in a regular push-up position like you were performing the standard Spiderman push-up. Take a "step" forward with your right hand and place it further in front of your body. Bend your arms and bring your left knee towards your left elbow as you lower yourself to the ground. Push yourself back up to your starting position, place your left foot back on the ground then take a "step" forward with your left hand and repeat the movement with your right leg.

DOWNWARD-FACING DOG INTO FORWARD-FACING DOG PUSH-UP

This fun twist to the famous yoga poses is a great exercise to help develop your chest, triceps, shoulders, core, glutes and hamstrings. Like the Spiderman push-up, this push-up variant also requires slow movements, extreme muscle control and balance.

Technique

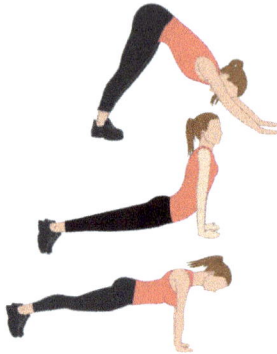

Start in the downward-facing dog position, where your buttocks are in the air, your back is straight, your core is engaged, and your hands and feet are flat on the ground. With a single movement, change into the forward-facing dog position by lifting your head and chest up and lowering your hips towards the ground until you are just holding your body above the ground with straight arms. Hold this position for a few seconds before tilting your upper body down into a push-up position. Perform a single push-up by bending your elbows and lowering yourself until your elbows are in line with your shoulders. Push yourself back up and once you have reached the top of your push-up, return to the downward-facing dog position.

This exercise can be deceivingly tiring, but it is a great exercise to do regularly because it incorporates both strength training and yoga components into one activity. If you are not flexible enough to put your feet flat on the ground during this exercise, don't worry – the flexibility will come (I still struggle to get my feet flat onto the ground with this one).

———

BURPEES

Burpees were created by a man named Royal H. Burpee who created the exercise as part of his thesis for his PhD in applied physiology; they didn't get their name because they can make you burp if you have had too many fluids beforehand, as many people believe. Burpees are a full body workout that targets nearly every muscle group in your body, and they were designed as a fundamental way to assess the overall fitness of an individual. They activate the muscles in your chest (particularly your pectoralis major), arms, back and shoulders in your upper half, as well as your abdominal muscles and quads, hamstrings and calves in your lower half.

Including burpees into your workout routine has a massive effect on your body. They make you burn loads of calories and are a perfect example of an exercise that produces the "afterburn" effect, increasing your metabolism and making you burn calories for hours after you have finished exercising. They are also great for cranking your heart rate up and improving your cardiovascular fitness. They might not be your favourite exercise, which is perfectly understandable as they can tire you out very quickly, but they are extremely effective.

Technique

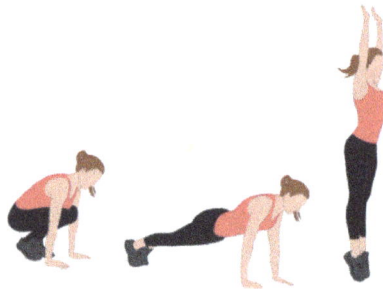

To perform this exercise, start by standing up straight with your arms by your side. Squat down and place your hands slightly wider than shoulder-width apart on the ground in front of you. Jump your legs out behind you so that you are now in a push-up position and perform a push-up. From here, jump to your feet and launch yourself upright into the air, stretching your arms above you and then land in the starting position. Repeat this movement as many times as you can.

If you start to feel tired and find yourself struggling to complete a full burpee, there are a few ways to make it easier while still working your entire body. Switch from a full push-up to a knee push-up and continue the exercise that way.

Alternatively, you can also cut down the exercise and only perform certain parts. For example, you could skip the push-up and lie flat on the ground before jumping up into the air, or you can skip the jump at the end and stand up straight after you have done your push-up. This still works many of the same muscles, just at a lower intensity.

———

5

BACK EXERCISES

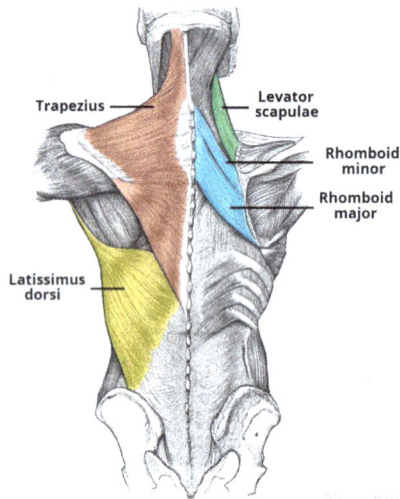

Photo of the superficial back muscles

There are many different muscles in the back, and they can all be found on separate layers. The most superficial layer contains the trapezius and the latissimus dorsi. The trapezius is a triangular-shaped muscle responsible for moving your shoulder blades, tilting and rotating your head as well as shrugging your shoulders. The latissimus dorsi is a large muscle that starts in the lower back and covers a broad area. It assists in many upper body movements and is primarily responsible for bringing your arm closer to your body, rotating your arm in towards your body and raising your arm out behind you. Slightly deeper to these muscles lie the rhomboid major and minor. These muscles help to rotate the shoulder blade and keep it attached to the rib cage. The levator scapulae is a strap-like muscle in the neck that helps to lift the shoulders.

An individual's back usually is one of the more neglected areas when it comes to working out. However, this is a rather dangerous area to neglect because it is more prone to injury the older you get. Fortunately, the back is targeted in many bodyweight exercises because the core muscles are activated, which has a direct effect on the back muscles themselves.

THE BENEFITS OF STRENGTHENING YOUR BACK

Similar to the chest muscles, the back muscles are involved in many upper body movements. Training the muscles in your back helps to make everyday tasks such as carrying objects and bending over to pick up items much easier, as well as helping to reduce the chances of injury later on in life. The middle of your back is an area that is very prone to osteoporotic fractures as you age and improving the strength of the back muscles can help to prevent this from occurring. The back muscles also have a powerful effect on our posture. As a society, we spend more time seated and hunched over than any previous generation due to technological advancements such as cars and laptops, meaning slouching and poor posture are very prevalent these days. Strengthening the muscles in the upper and middle back can help pull the shoulders back to their correct position.

One of the additional benefits of exercising your back is that it can have a direct effect on reducing the recurrence of tension headaches. The muscles in the back influence the muscles in the head due to their neighbouring attachment points. For example, the trapezius attaches to the base of the skull. If this muscle is in a spasm, which it regularly is because of the amount of time people spend hunched over and slouching, it can cause the sudden onset of an inexplicable headache. Releasing the tension in this muscle through exercising, stretching, or massaging your back muscles can significantly reduce the severity of the headache.

———

WIDE OVERHAND PULL-UP/OVERHAND INVERTED ROW

Wide grip pull-ups are one of the most effective workouts that you can attempt to target your back, chest, shoulders, arms and core muscles. Pull-ups use an overhand grip (where your palms face away from you) and focus more on training your latissimus dorsi. Similar to the underhand chin-up, they look much easier than they actually are. However, the wide-grip pull-up is much harder than standard pull-ups because your hands are spread further apart, making your latissimus dorsi work even harder. The further apart your hands are, the more challenging the exercise is. It is another excellent exercise that can be used as a way to monitor your progress, and the more you practice it, the more reps you will be able to do.

Wide Overhand Pull-up

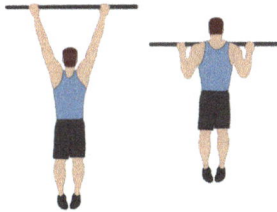

To perform a wide overhand pull-up, reach your arms up and grasp the bar (or other raised surface) with your hands positioned wider than your body and your palms facing away from you. If you have placed your arms correctly, your body should look like it is in a "Y-shape." From here, bend your arms at the elbow and pull yourself up until your chin has passed the bar. Have your legs positioned slightly in front of your body and point your toes towards the ground with your knees nice and straight. Make sure to keep your back straight, your chest up and engage your core to help keep your body stable. Once your chin has passed the bar, hold this position for a few seconds before slowly lowering yourself back down until your arms are straight.

When it comes to gripping the bar with your fingers, the part of your hand which you are using matters a lot. Some people grip the bar with the tips of their fingers resting over the top of the bar, making their hand into a claw or a hook shape. On the other hand, others prefer to grip the bar deeper into the hand with their palms. You will be able to perform more pull-ups if you grip the bar using that claw position (with your fingers resting on top of the bar), but this can cause problems in the long run. When you do pull-ups with your hands in this position, it puts lots of stress on the deep muscles and tendons which travel down the forearm and attach to the inside of the elbow. Repeatedly doing pull-ups using this hand position can cause a condition known as medial epicondylitis (also known as golfer's elbow) which causes those tendons to become swollen and painful. It is much better to grip the bar using your palm with your fingers fully wrapped around the bar. Your elbows will thank you later.

Also, when it comes to pulling your body up to the bar, make sure to focus on squeezing the bar with your hand, particularly your ring and pinky fingers. This might sound a little odd, but the reason for this is because these two fingers are the weakest in your grip. If you focus on squeezing the bar with these two weaker fingers, the rest of the fingers in the grip will be stronger and you'll have a much stronger force going down into the bar, helping to pull your body up.

Overhand Inverted Row

Similar to the underhand chin-up, this exercise is much easier to do with a pull-up bar. However, if you don't have a bar, here are a few ways to work the same muscles.

If you have a park nearby with some raised bars or some low tree branches, then you can use those and apply the same technique as I have described above. Just remember to make sure they are sturdy enough to support your weight. If you don't have any of those, you can do inverted rows with an overhand grip.

To perform this exercise, you need a sturdy table (one that isn't going to break or flip over if you apply weight to it) or a low railing. Position yourself under the table or railing and lie with your chest directly underneath it. Grasp it with your hands either shoulder-width apart or wider than your body (depending on whether you want to perform wide grip inverted rows or not) using an overhand grip. Keep your whole body straight, engage your core and then pull yourself up to the table/railing as high as you can whilst keeping your heels on the ground. Hold this position for a few seconds before lowering yourself back down to the starting position. You can make this exercise harder by raising your feet onto a chair and performing the inverted row that way.

———

DOLPHIN KICK

The dolphin kick (also known as reverse hyperextensions) is an exercise that works your lower back, glutes and hamstrings all at the same time. The main movement involved in the exercise is extension of the hips, which is a movement that features a lot when running, jumping or kicking, and if you aren't very flexible, these can be much harder to do. It is also a great exercise to help improve or prevent lower back pain. Lower back pain commonly occurs when the muscles of the lower back, glutes and hamstrings are weak or if they are injured during exercises or movements which can put a lot of strain on your lower back, such as deadlifts or lifting weights that are too heavy. The dolphin kick doesn't put any stress on the lower back and allows you to strengthen these muscles without risking injury.

Technique

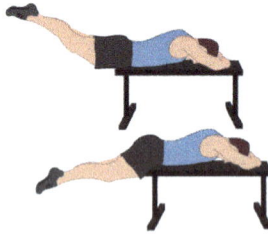

Lie on your front on a firm raised surface such as an exercise bench or your bed (as long as it isn't too soft) with your hips on the edge and your feet touching the ground behind you. Keep your arms out in front of you and if you need to, feel free to hold on to something to help give you some support and stability. Contract your glutes and hamstrings to slowly raise your legs behind you until they are in a straight line. Hold this position for a few seconds then slowly lower your legs back down to the ground.

The higher the surface that you are lying on, the more difficult the exercise will be. If you want to make the exercise more challenging, gradually increase the height of the surface you are lying on.

———

SUPERMAN

This exercise is one of the best to train the muscles in your lower back and help relieve any long-standing back pain you may have. As well as working the muscles in your lower back, it strengthens your latissimus dorsi, glutes and hamstrings too, making it a great exercise to work your entire posterior chain (the muscles that lie along the back of your body).

Technique

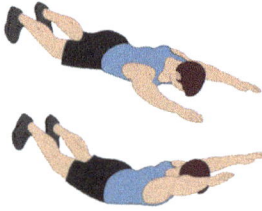

Lie face down and place your arms out in front of you, so your hands and elbows are flat on the ground. Inhale deeply and lift your arms and chest off the floor while you contract your glutes and hamstrings to lift your legs off the ground. You want to try and make a U-shape with your body and get as much curve in your back as you can. Remember to engage your core during this exercise by squeezing your abdominal muscles. If you have done this movement correctly, you should look like the Man of Steel flying through the sky. Try to hold this position for as long as you can.

Although this exercise may seem easy, it can turn out to be quite tiring. When you are just starting, you might only be able to hold it for a few seconds, but this will improve with time.

———

BACK WIDOW

The back widow is a great exercise to help target your trapezius, rhomboids and the posterior portion of your deltoid. Strengthening these muscles can help prevent your shoulders and chest hunching forward by reducing any muscle imbalances between your chest muscles and the muscles in the middle of your back. It is basically a push-up that works your back and shoulders instead of your chest and arms, and it is extremely effective at building up the muscles in your back.

Technique

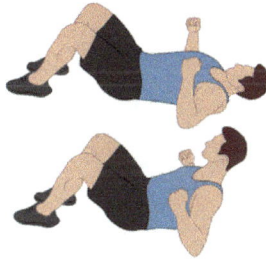

Start by lying on your back with your elbows at a 45-degree angle away from your sides. Point your forearms up to the ceiling and place your feet flat on the ground. Push your elbows into the ground to lift your upper back into the air while keeping your feet flat on the ground. Try to hold this position for a few seconds as that will help keep your back muscles contracting for longer and ensure you haven't lifted yourself off the ground just using momentum.

If you want to make this exercise even more challenging, you can attempt raised back widows. Grab two chairs, benches, stools etc. and position them either side of your body. Place your elbows in the middle of the raised surface at 90-degrees, so your upper body is in a U-shape. Extend your legs out in front of you with your heels on the ground, or if you want to make the exercise slightly easier, place your feet flat on the ground with your knees bent. From here, lift your hips slightly off the ground and then drive through your elbows to push your body up until it is in a straight line. Hold this position for a few seconds and then slowly lower yourself back down.

———

SCAPULAR PUSH-UP

This push-up variant is a great exercise to target the muscles around the shoulder blade, specifically the rhomboids, levator scapulae, serratus anterior and your pectoralis minor. Strengthening these muscles can help improve the natural movements of the shoulder blade. While this might not sound too important, your shoulder blades are involved in many upper body movements, especially in sports that require an extensive range of motion such as golf and tennis. Strengthening these muscles can also help to improve your posture and maintaining the plank position while performing this small movement can help develop your core strength too.

Technique

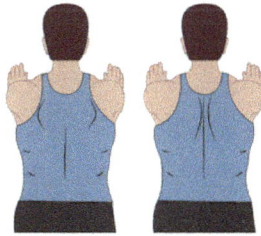

To perform this exercise, get into a high plank position with your hands shoulder-width apart and your feet together. Keep your back straight, engage your core and don't let your hips sag down. Keep your arms straight (elbows locked) and try to pinch your shoulder blades together. Remember you are not doing a traditional push-up; only a small amount of movement is required to pinch your shoulder blades together. Hold this position for a few seconds then push your shoulder blades back to the starting position.

If you find you are struggling to maintain the plank position or you struggle to keep your arms straight, try performing the scapular push-up from your knees instead (like you were performing a knee push-up). It is more important to focus on the motion of pinching your shoulder blades together rather than maintaining the plank position.

———

6

CORE AND ABDOMINAL EXERCISES

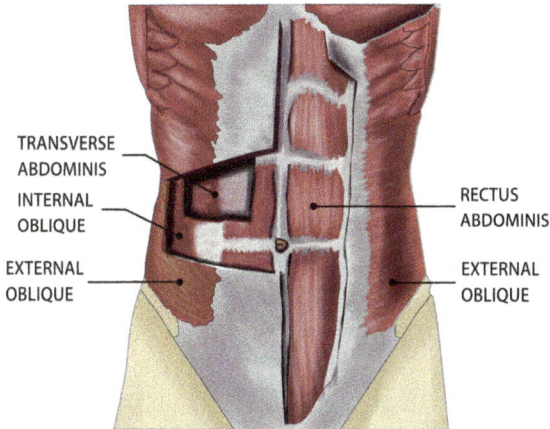

Photo of the abdominal muscles

The abdominal muscles are a popular area of the body that people love to work on. There are several muscles in the abdomen, and they can be found on different layers. The most superficial layer contains the external obliques which can be found on the front and side of your abdomen. Underneath the external obliques lie the internal obliques and the rectus abdominis muscles in the center of your abdomen. The rectus abdominis are the most well-known muscles in the abdomen and are also known as the "six-pack" muscles. Underneath the internal obliques lie the transverse abdominis. These muscles wrap around the spine to help keep it stable and protected.

However, the abdominal muscles are often mistaken to be the core muscles, but this isn't the case. The core muscles extend way beyond the abdominal muscles and comprise of as many as 35 different groups of muscles. Many of these muscles are hidden deeper into the torso. The major muscles of the core include the abdominal muscles, the pelvic floor muscles, erector spinae (the muscles that run along the length of the spine), quadratus lumborum (the deepest abdominal muscle either side of your lower spine), the hip flexors and the diaphragm.

Your hip flexors are muscles that aren't often discussed, but they are very important. The main hip flexors in the body are the iliopsoas (made up of the iliacus and psoas muscles), sartorius (fun fact – the longest muscle in your body) and rectus femoris (the largest and most superficial quadriceps muscle). These muscles are involved in many upper leg movements such as lifting your thigh upwards, moving your leg side to side, as well as tilting your torso forward and keeping your lower body stable.

When you think of your core, it is beneficial to think of it as a central link between your upper and lower body. When you move, the essential motions either originate from your core muscles or pass through them. Therefore, they are extremely important muscles, and that is why it is necessary to strengthen them.

Fortunately, practically all bodyweight exercises directly or indirectly target your core. When it comes to defining your abs, focusing on core exercises is one of the best methods to define them. This is because you are building the strength of these muscles from the inside out, making the noticeable effects apparent in a much shorter period of time. You may be surprised (or relieved) to see that there are no versions of sit-ups or crunches in this section of the book. Instead, we are going to focus on workouts that will strengthen the entirety of your trunk. This will define your abs and strengthen the other muscles in your core.

THE BENEFITS OF STRENGTHENING YOUR ABS AND CORE

As well as the aesthetics of how defined abs look, there are many other reasons why it is beneficial to strengthen your core. Your core muscles are involved in nearly everything you do. Whether you are putting on your shoes, getting dressed or even sitting upright at a desk typing on a computer, you are using your core muscles. The core muscles help to keep your body stable, allowing you to move in every direction, as well as ensuring you remain balanced and upright. Weak core muscles can increase your chances of falling over and injuring yourself. Lower back pain is a very prevalent and sometimes debilitating issue that can affect people as they age, and the chances of this occurring can be reduced by including core workouts into your weekly routine.

Almost every sporting activity involves the use of your core, from golf and tennis to swimming, basketball and horse riding. Weak core muscles can prevent people from doing these activities and reduce the quality of their sporting performances. Your core also has a strong effect on your posture and can help reduce the harsh effects of wear and tear on your spine. A weak core can affect your body in a multitude of ways and neglecting these muscles can significantly affect you in the future.

———

PLANK

One of the most effective core workouts that you can perform is the basic plank. This exercise targets the rectus abdominis, the obliques, the serratus anterior, the triceps, the lower back, quadriceps and the hip flexor muscles. As you can see, an incredible number of muscles are activated by an exercise that basically requires you to stay still.

A common misconception about the plank is that it is effective at targeting the glutes and you are often instructed to squeeze them while you are holding the plank position. However, this actually doesn't have any effect on your glutes. This is because there is no resistance being applied to them when you are planking. Your glutes aren't responsible for maintaining the plank position in any way. If you were lying on the ground and you contracted your gluteal muscles, you would actually be pushing your body further into the ground and not up into the air. In reality, it is your hip flexors that lift your body into the air, and the plank position is maintained with help from your other core muscles. However, your gluteal muscles are targeted in the reverse plank which will be discussed next.

Planking is also an exercise that can help increase your metabolism due to the large number of muscles that are activated during the exercise, allowing you to burn lots of calories.

Technique

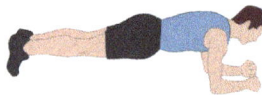

Lie down on your front, place your elbows underneath your shoulders and rest your forearms on the ground. Extend your legs out behind you about hip-width apart and lift your body off the ground, balancing on your forearms and toes. Make sure to engage your core, keep your hips level and look down to the floor to help keep your spine in a neutral position. Maintain your straight posture and hold this position for as long as you can.

In the beginning stages of planking, you might start to feel your muscles struggling and shaking rather quickly. Try to hold the position for as long as you can but stop once you begin to notice your form going downhill. It is much more beneficial to hold the plank for less time with proper form, rather than force yourself to continue with poor form. Start off aiming for around 10 seconds and then gradually increase your target as you get better.

———

REVERSE PLANK

The reverse plank is an exercise that is often under-utilized, and it is very similar to the regular plank, but it focusses more on the muscles on the back of the body instead of the front. It is a great exercise for targeting the core muscles as well as the shoulders, arms, glutes and hamstrings. While it is strengthening these muscles, it also stretches the muscles in the chest and shoulders, helping to prevent you from developing a hunched posture. It is another excellent exercise that can help prevent back pain occurring by strengthening the lower back muscles without placing any pressure on the spine.

Technique

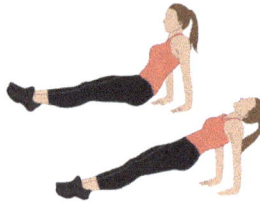

Start from a seated position on the floor, extend your legs out in front of you and place your hands slightly wider than shoulder-width apart behind you with your fingers facing forward. Engage your core and raise your hips until your body is straight and you are supporting your body weight with your heels and straight arms. Make sure to drop your shoulders down so they are not hunched near your ears and keep your head in line with your body to avoid straining your neck. Hold this position for as long as you can before slowly lowering yourself back down to your seated position.

If you want to make this exercise even more challenging, try slowly raising and lowering each leg. This helps to work your glutes and hamstrings even more than the standard reverse plank.

For a more advanced version, try the standard reverse plank (without raising your legs) but support your body using your forearms to keep your body straight. If you have mastered that, add in the leg raises to challenge yourself more.

———

SEATED AB CIRCLES

Seated ab circles are an extremely effective exercise that targets your abdominal muscles and your hip flexors. It might look easy, but it is an exercise that is deceivingly difficult and will have your abs burning in a short space of time (in a good way, of course).

Technique

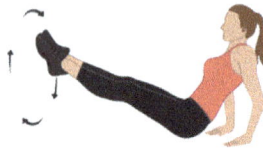

To perform this exercise, sit down on the ground with your legs extended out in front of you. Place your hands out to the side of your body with your palms flat on the floor. Keep your legs together, point your toes, lift your legs off the ground and lean back slightly, using your hands for support. Move your legs clockwise in circles and squeeze your core when your legs are at the top of the rotation. Make sure to keep your upper body stationary; only your legs should be moving. Keep repeating these circles without letting your legs touch the ground; the higher your lift your legs, the more your abdominal muscles will be working. Once you have completed the circles with your legs rotating clockwise, repeat the exercise with your legs rotating anticlockwise.

If you want to make this exercise slightly easier, start by making smaller circles with your legs and gradually increasing the circle size as time goes on. If you are feeling brave and want to make the exercise more challenging, try adding some weights to your ankles such as a bag with a heavy item in it.

DRUNKEN MOUNTAIN CLIMBERS

Regular mountain climbers are a great exercise to target your abdominals, glutes, legs, arms and shoulder muscles, while also causing your heart rate to skyrocket up. Drunken mountain climbers take this to a new level, putting more emphasis on your oblique muscles by adding in a twisting movement to the exercise. Despite the name, I wouldn't recommend actually getting drunk to do this exercise as that will make it significantly harder.

Technique

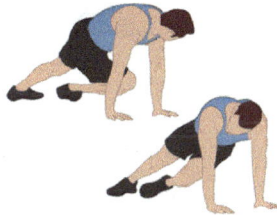

To perform drunken mountain climbers, get into a high plank position with your arms shoulder-width apart and your legs extended out behind you. Keep your back straight, engage your core and keep your wrists directly below your shoulders to help activate your shoulder muscles. Bring your left knee across your body and try to touch your right elbow, rotating your body to the right as you do so. Slightly pause as your knee reaches your elbow to ensure your abdominal muscles are fully contracting, then bring your left knee back across your body and return to your original position. Repeat this on the other side by trying to bring your right knee in to touch your left elbow, rotating your body to the left. Continue this movement and alternate the leg you use each time.

———

SCISSOR KICKS

Scissor kicks are mainly a lower abdominal exercise which target your core muscles as well as your glutes, quads and leg adductors. Your leg adductors are the muscles that lie on the inside of your thigh and bring your leg in closer to your body.

Technique

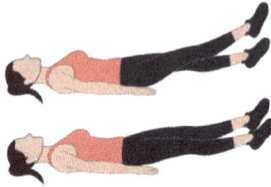

To perform this exercise, lie flat on your back with your legs extended and place your arms out to the side with your palms flat on the floor. Alternatively, place your hands underneath your buttocks if you want to support your back. Engage your core and lift your legs off the ground, slightly bending your knees to take some pressure off your back. Cross your right leg over the top while your left leg crosses underneath. Then repeat this by crossing your left leg over your right leg. If done correctly, it should look like your legs are doing a scissor action over the top of each other. Repeatedly alternate this movement with each leg whilst keeping your legs off the ground. Try to keep the movement of your legs rhythmical and controlled. Don't go too fast (or too furious).

———

HANGING LEG RAISE/CHAIR LEG RAISE

The hanging leg raise is an advanced exercise, and it is one of the best you can do to target the abdominal muscles and hip flexors. This exercise uses the weight of your legs as resistance, making the movement harder. It also works the muscles in your arms, shoulders and back to a lesser degree as you hold your body weight up off the ground. If you don't have a bar or any other suitable surface to hang from, I will show you an alternative exercise you can do instead.

Hanging Leg Raise

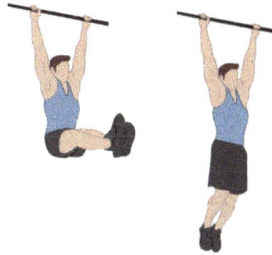

To perform this exercise, grasp a bar (or other stable surface above your head) with your hands shoulder-width apart using an overhand grip (palms facing away from you). Keep your back straight, engage your core and slowly raise your legs from the hips until they are parallel to the ground. Not everyone will be flexible enough to have their legs entirely straight at 90-degrees; if this is the case for you, slightly bend your knees to help lift your legs until they are parallel. Once you have raised your legs, hold that position for a few seconds before slowly lowering your legs down to your starting position.

Make sure you focus on contracting your abdominal muscles and hip flexors to bend your legs. A common mistake people make is swinging their legs and using their body's momentum to help raise their legs to 90-degrees. This will help raise your legs, but it won't be working your core muscles. There are two effective ways to help prevent your legs from swinging.

Firstly, don't have your legs hanging straight down. Similar to the pull-up, have your legs positioned slightly in front of your body as this will partially contract the abdominal muscles and provide some stabilization. Secondly, keep your shoulder blades back and down. If you hunch your shoulders, your upper body will be less stable and more likely to swing. This simple adjustment to the positioning of your shoulder blades will help keep your upper body more stable. If you make these two changes and focus on performing slow and controlled movements, you will work your abdominal muscles and hip flexors much more.

If you want to make this exercise even more challenging, try raising your legs until they are about shoulder height. This will help target your rectus abdominis even more.

Chair Leg Raise

If you don't have a pull-up bar or any other suitable surface, you can still perform this exercise. Grab two sturdy chairs and put them on either side of your body with the backs of the chairs next to your arms. Place your hands on the top of the chairs and extend your arms to lift your body until your feet are dangling off the ground. From here, position your feet slightly in front of your body and engage your core to lift your legs up to 90-degrees (or higher if you can manage it). Hold this position for a few seconds before slowly lowering yourself back down to the ground.

If you plan on trying this method, please make sure the chairs are on a stable surface and they are strong enough not to break or topple. It might be beneficial to place something heavy on the flat cushion part of the chairs to make them less likely to topple over.

———

7

GLUTE EXERCISES

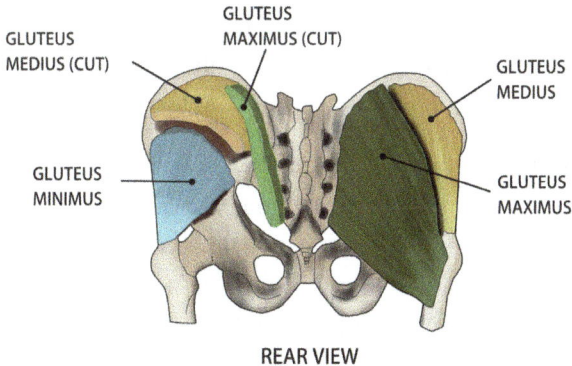

GLUTEUS
MEDIUS (CUT)

GLUTEUS
MAXIMUS (CUT)

GLUTEUS
MEDIUS

GLUTEUS
MINIMUS

GLUTEUS
MAXIMUS

REAR VIEW

Photo of the gluteal muscles from the rear

The gluteal muscles are usually an area that is neglected by male exercisers, which is unfortunate because there are many benefits to having strong glutes. Fortunately, many of the leg exercises that people partake in actively exercise the gluteal muscles.

The gluteal muscles are made up of 3 individual muscles. The most superficial muscle is the gluteus maximus which forms the round shape of the buttocks. It is the largest muscle in the body and also one of the strongest. Its primary function is to extend the leg at the hip, an action that commonly occurs when we walk, run or jump. Underneath the gluteus maximus lies the gluteus medius and gluteus minimus. These two muscles act as pelvic stabilizers, keeping the pelvis in place when we move. They also rotate the leg inwards and move the leg out to the side.

THE BENEFITS OF STRENGTHENING YOUR GLUTES

Increasing the strength of your glutes can help make everyday activities such as running, lifting objects and climbing stairs much more manageable. When the gluteal muscles are weak, the stronger latissimus dorsi and hip flexors can pull your torso, shoulders and pelvis into an abnormal position, which can result in pain and poor posture. Therefore, strengthening your glutes can have a significant impact on your posture.

The gluteal muscles have a large role in supporting the lower back, and if these muscles are weak, they may not be able to carry out their role of extending the leg effectively. When this happens, the body relies on other muscles to carry out that role, and these muscles can become overloaded, causing pain and compression in the lower back, hips and knees. Also, because they have a role in stabilizing the pelvis, weak glutes can cause the body's alignment to fall out of position. This increases the likelihood of injuries such as anterior cruciate ligament tears in the knee, tendonitis (notably of the Achilles tendon in your heel) and shin splints. Training your glutes can help reduce the chances of any injuries like these occurring as well as preventing and relieving pain in the lower back, hips and knees.

However, one of the most valuable benefits of strengthening your glutes is the effect it can have on your athletic performance. The gluteal muscles are responsible for many movements in the lower

GLUTE EXERCISES | 97

limb that are invaluable in sports. Running, jumping and changing direction all involve the gluteal muscles. Athletes who train their glutes have a lot more explosive power available to them than those who don't.

———

SINGLE-LEG GLUTE BRIDGE

The single-leg glute bridge is a progression of the standard glute bridge, and it is an effective exercise that primarily targets your glutes and hamstrings. It also works the core muscles, notably your abdominal and lower back muscles. It is a slow exercise that works very well as part of the final stages of your workout routine after you have completed higher-intensity exercises.

Technique

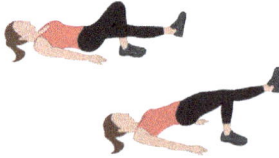

To perform this exercise, start by lying on the ground with your hands placed by your sides and your feet flat. Straighten one of your legs out in front of you, engage your core and glutes and lift your hips towards the ceiling until you form a straight bridge shape with your body. Hold this position for a few seconds before slowly lowering yourself back down to the ground and repeating the exercise with the other leg.

Make sure to keep your back straight when you are in the bridge position; you are using your gluteal muscles to raise yourself into the air, not the muscles in your back. You also want to keep your hips level when you are performing this exercise. If you find that one side of your hips keeps sagging or rotating down, try the standard glute bridge, where you perform this movement with both feet on the ground instead of straightening one of your legs, until you are strong enough to perform this exercise.

———

SLICK FLOOR BRIDGE CURLS

Slick floor bridge curls are a variation of the standard glute bridge that is effective at targeting both your glutes and hamstrings by making them work together. Your hamstrings are responsible for sliding your feet back in towards your body and maintaining the bridge position throughout the exercise helps ensure that your glutes are the main muscles targeted. Other than yourself, you need two things for this exercise: a pair of socks and a slick floor that you can slide on such as a tiled or shiny wooden floor. If your house has rooms with carpet and a smooth floor next to each other, for example, if your living room has carpet and your hallway has a slick floor, you can rest your upper body on the carpet to stop it sliding and have your lower body on the slick surface.

Technique

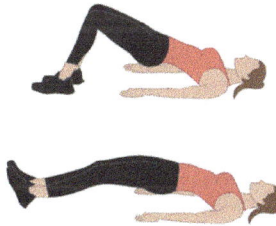

To perform this exercise, lie on your back on the slick surface, place your hands out to the side and place your feet flat on the ground. Get into the bridge position by lifting your hips until your body is in a straight line from your head to your knees. From here, extend your legs and slide your feet along the slick surface until you are resting on your heels. Keep your core and glutes engaged to keep your body raised off the ground as you straighten your legs. Then slide your heels back in towards your body until you are back in that original bridge position with your feet flat on the floor. If you want to perform these exercises with trainers on, all you need to do is put a towel down underneath your feet and use them to slide the towel along the floor.

If you find this exercise challenging, start by extending your legs a small distance and then increase this as you get stronger. If you want to make this exercise more challenging, you can try the "squeeze' slick floor bridge curl. All you need is a foam roller, rolled up towel or similar household item which you hold between your legs as you slide your feet across the floor. This will help target the adductor muscles on the inside of your leg that pull your legs closer to your body.

———

BULGARIAN SPLIT SQUAT

The Bulgarian split squat is a variation of the traditional squat, and it is one of the best exercises for targeting the glutes, hamstrings, quads and calf muscles. It also works to improve your core muscle strength and balance as you lower and raise your body using just one leg. As you are working on one side at a time, this exercise helps to improve any muscle imbalances between your left and right side, allowing your body to maintain its correct alignment and reduce the likelihood of injuries occurring. You can perform this exercise using just your body weight, or you can add in more resistance by holding household items such as water bottles as weights once you have become more proficient at the exercise.

Technique

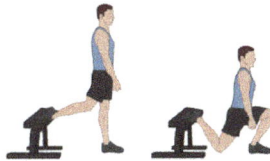

Stand in front of a raised surface such as a bench, chair or sofa, with your feet positioned about shoulder-width apart. Lift your right foot and place it on top of the raised surface behind you. You need to position your left foot far enough forward so you can squat comfortably but not too close so that you lift the heel of your left foot off the ground as you lower your body; adjust the positioning of your foot until it feels comfortable. Engage your core, keep your back straight and slightly angle your upper body forward, then bend your left knee to lower yourself down to the ground. Go as low as you comfortably can, aiming to stop when your left thigh is parallel to the ground. Hold this position for a few seconds before driving your left foot into the ground to push yourself back up to the starting position. Repeat this movement on the other side. If you find that the stretch in your

102 | HOME WORKOUTS

legs and groin is too intense, try performing the exercise on a lower surface.

A common mistake with the Bulgarian split squat (and squat exercises in general) is that people let their knee roll further forward than their toes. Make sure your knee doesn't roll too far forward as this can put pressure on the knee joint and cause issues later on in life. Hold on to a wall for balance if you need to.

———

HIP THRUSTS

Hip thrusts are renowned for being one of the best exercises to target and build your glutes, as well as working the hamstrings, quads and core muscles. It is especially beneficial for improving the hip mobility of individuals who spend much of their day sitting at a desk, as it involves putting the lower body through a large range of motion. You will quickly see why this is an exercise that is becoming more and more popular.

Technique

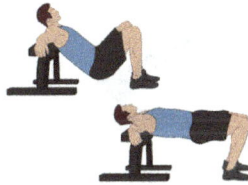

To perform this exercise, sit on the floor with a raised surface behind you, such as a bench or sofa, and place your feet flat on the ground. Try to position your feet far enough away from your buttocks so that there's a 90-degree angle at your knee when your body is straight, otherwise you might put some strain on your knees. Lean back and rest your upper back on the raised surface and extend your arms out to the side along the length of the raised surface. From here, keep your back straight, engage your core and glutes and drive your feet into the ground, lifting your hips to the ceiling until your body is straight. Hold this position for a few seconds (while contracting your gluteal muscles) before lowering yourself back down to the starting position. When you are lowering your body back down, don't go so low that your buttocks touch the floor. Keep them raised off the floor to help ensure your glutes are working through the whole exercise.

If you want to make this exercise even harder, try performing it using just one leg to challenge your lower body even more.

SIDE LEG RAISE

This exercise is great for targeting your gluteal muscles, notably your gluteus medius and gluteus minimus. These muscles are responsible for stabilizing your pelvis and for leg abduction, which is when you move your leg out to the side and away from the midline of your body.

Technique

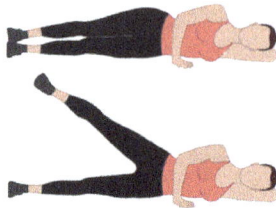

To perform this exercise, lie on the floor on your left side, with your body in a straight line. Place your right hand either on your hip or on the floor to keep you balanced. Keep your back straight, engage your core and lift your right leg towards the ceiling. Hold this position for a few seconds at the top of the movement and then slowly bring your leg back down towards your body. When bringing your leg back down, don't let it rest on your other leg; try to keep it slightly raised above your other leg as this will help ensure your glutes are working throughout the whole movement.

A common mistake that occurs with this exercise is that people perform this movement with their toes pointing up towards the ceiling. When the toe is pointing up to the ceiling, the leg is externally rotated, meaning that the hip flexors are now the primary muscles performing the movement. An easy fix to sort this is to try and angle your toes so they are pointing down towards the floor. This change in positioning causes the leg to internally rotate and ensures the gluteus medius and minimus are doing the work to lift the leg.

Another common mistake people make is that they lift their leg in more of a diagonal direction away from the body instead of straight up towards the ceiling. This happens because the quads are often stronger than the hamstrings and as the leg is raised, it can creep forward. Try to make sure you are lifting your leg straight out to the side to target your glutes fully.

———

8

LEG EXERCISES

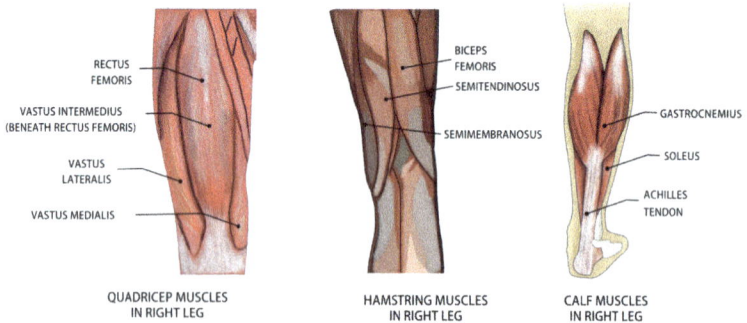

RECTUS FEMORIS

VASTUS INTERMEDIUS (BENEATH RECTUS FEMORIS)

VASTUS LATERALIS

VASTUS MEDIALIS

BICEPS FEMORIS

SEMITENDINOSUS

SEMIMEMBRANOSUS

GASTROCNEMIUS

SOLEUS

ACHILLES TENDON

QUADRICEP MUSCLES IN RIGHT LEG

HAMSTRING MUSCLES IN RIGHT LEG

CALF MUSCLES IN RIGHT LEG

Photo of quadriceps (left), hamstring (middle) and calf muscles (right) in the right leg

Anatomy-wise, the leg is divided into roughly four main muscle groups: the gluteal muscles in the buttocks, the quadriceps at the front of the upper leg, the hamstring muscles at the back of the upper leg and the calves at the back of the lower leg.

The quadriceps are made up of four individual muscles: the rectus femoris (the big boy at the top of your thigh) and the vastus lateralis, vastus intermedius and vastus medialis which all lie underneath the rectus femoris. These four muscles make up the vast majority of the thigh and are some of the strongest muscles in the body. The main function of these muscles is to lift the thigh upwards and straighten the leg at the knee joint.

The hamstring muscles lie on the back of the thigh and are made up of three muscles: the biceps femoris, semitendinosus and semimembranosus. The main function of these muscles is to extend the leg at the hip and bend the knee joint.

Moving further down the back of the leg lies the calf muscles. The calf is made up of three muscles: the gastrocnemius, which is the most superficial muscle, and the soleus and plantaris which lie just underneath it. These muscles are responsible for pointing your toes and lifting your body onto the tips of your toes.

THE BENEFITS OF STRENGTHENING YOUR LEGS

Strengthening the muscles in your lower body is beneficial for a multitude of reasons. You rely on your legs for movements like walking, climbing stairs and running, and strengthening them now can help give you more independence later on in life.

Lower limb injuries such as ankle and knee injuries are common, especially for those who play sport. Training the muscles in your legs can help make them stronger and help improve any muscle imbalances you may have. Also, the muscles in your lower half are some of the largest in your body, and larger muscles burn more calories than smaller ones. Regularly strengthening your legs will help increase your metabolism, allowing you to burn more calories and develop even more muscle growth.

SQUATS

Squats are one of the best workouts to target nearly every muscle in your lower body. They train your quads, glutes, hamstrings and calves and are perfect if you want to improve the strength and tone of your lower half as well as improving your overall fitness. It is an efficient and effective exercise, even when you are solely using your body weight.

Technique

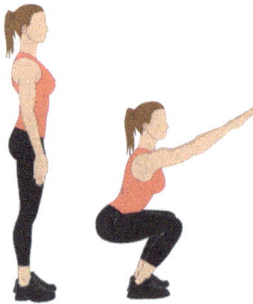

To perform this exercise, place your feet about hip-width apart and angle them slightly outwards. Keep your back straight, engage your core and bend your knees to lower yourself down towards the ground. Try to keep your chest up and don't let your upper body lean forward. Keep lowering your body until your thighs are parallel to the ground and don't let your knees roll forward and pass the line of your toes. Hold this position for a few seconds then drive through your heels to push yourself back up to a standing position. Your hand positioning isn't too crucial for this exercise. Some people prefer to extend their arms out in front of them while others prefer to bring their hands in together. Choose what feels most comfortable for you.

A common mistake people make when doing squats is that they don't lower themselves down far enough towards the ground. It is important to try to lower yourself until your thighs are parallel to the ground as this will ensure you are fully activating the muscles in your legs. However, only go as low as you comfortably can. If you feel any discomfort in your knees or hips, this indicates that this level is your endpoint. There's no point in forcing it and risking injury. Start off going as low as you can and gradually try to increase this as time goes on.

If you want to make this exercise more interesting, you can try these two variations: the launch squat and the sumo squat.

The **launch squat** is great because it targets the same muscles as the basic squat with the added benefit of it being a powerful aerobic exercise. This exercise requires you to exert your muscles in a short period of time while also causing your heart rate to spike up. It is similar to the standard squat, where you keep your back straight, bend your knees and lower yourself until your thighs are parallel to the ground (or as close as you comfortably can go). However, instead of straightening your legs and returning to your original standing position, launch yourself into the air after each squat and land softly with your knees bent, ready to go straight into the next repetition. If you are just starting, try a low jump first and then gradually increase the height as you get fitter.

The **sumo squat** also targets the same muscles as the standard squat, but the wider stance places more focus on the adductor muscles in your inner thigh. Stand with your feet set wider than shoulder-width apart and angle your toes out at a 45-degree angle (doing this will help take the strain off your knees). Keep your back straight, engage your core and try to lower yourself down until your thighs are parallel to the ground. Hold this position for a few seconds before returning to your original position.

———

SINGLE-LEG CALF RAISES

When it comes to lower body exercises, people tend to focus more on their glutes, hamstrings and quads, often neglecting their calves. However, strengthening these muscles can reduce the chances of ankle injuries, increase jumping height and improve overall athletic performance. Thankfully, single-leg calf raises are one of the best exercises for building these muscles. The best place to perform this exercise is on one of the steps that you probably have around your home, and they can be performed using your body weight or by holding some weights from around the house. I would recommend holding a large filled water bottle or a dumbbell if you have it.

Technique

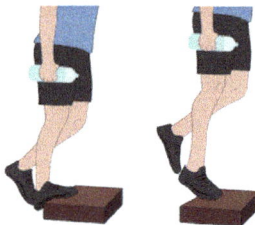

To start, place the ball of your right foot on an elevated surface and cross your left foot behind your right foot, resting it on your heel to keep yourself stable. If you are using a weight, make sure to hold it in the hand on the side you are working; when you are working your right calf, hold the weight in your right hand. Hold a wall for support (if you need to) and make sure your right knee is straight as this helps to fully engage the gastrocnemius muscle of the calf. From here, slowly drop down until you can feel a stretch in your right calf and hold that position for a few seconds. Then drive through the ball of your right foot and lift your heel into the air as high as you can, squeezing your right calf at the top of the movement. Hold this position for a few seconds then lower yourself back down to the starting position. Repeat this movement on your left side.

This exercise is extremely effective at strengthening the calf muscles. However, the calf muscles don't always act according to the same principles as other muscles. Calf muscle growth and development has a genetic aspect – some people are genetically predisposed to have smaller calves, no matter how hard they train them. If you fall into this category, don't fret. Lean calf muscles can be just as strong as larger ones. Size isn't everything.

———

REVERSE LUNGE WITH FRONT KICK

This exercise is an amalgamation of the reverse lunge and high kick exercises, and it targets the hamstrings, quads, hip flexors, glutes and core muscles. It helps to improve any muscle imbalances between your right and left legs and improves your balance and coordination. You may find yourself wobbling initially, but over time, your balance will improve. This exercise does require more free space as you will be kicking your leg out, so make sure there is nothing breakable or fragile nearby.

Technique

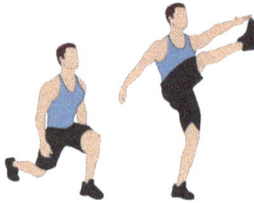

Start this exercise by standing with your feet about shoulder-width apart and your toes pointing straight. Keep your back straight, engage your core and move your right leg out behind you while simultaneously bending your left knee and lowering yourself down towards the ground. Keep lowering yourself until your left thigh is parallel to the ground and your right knee is hovering just above the ground. Hold this position for a few seconds then drive through the ground with your left foot to bring yourself back up to a standing position, whilst swinging your right leg forward and kicking in front of you as you rise. Bring your right leg back down and swing it behind your body, ready to go into the next lunge. Perform all the repetitions on the right side of your body then repeat with your left side.

SPLIT SQUAT JUMP

This is an explosive exercise that primarily targets the quadriceps but also works the hamstrings, glutes and calves. Not only will it cause your heart rate to skyrocket up and give you a very satisfying burn in your quads, it will also help improve your balance, stability and overall body control.

Technique

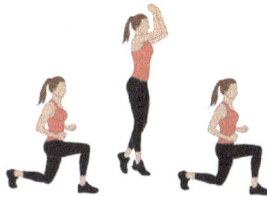

To perform this exercise, stand with your feet about shoulder-width apart and your arms by your side. Keep your back straight, engage your core and lunge forward with your right foot, lowering your body until your right thigh is parallel to the ground and your left knee is hovering above the ground. Make sure your right knee doesn't roll further forward than your toes. From here, drive through your right foot and jump into the air. Switch the positioning of your legs and land in the lunge position, this time with your left foot forward and your right leg behind. Drive through your left foot and jump into the air, switching the positioning of your legs again. Repeat this movement.

If you want to make this exercise even more challenging, grab some dumbbells (if you have them) or some filled water bottles/bags of flour and hold them by your side as you perform this exercise.

———

PISTOL SQUAT

Now before you think you are going to get away without any challenging exercises in this chapter, this one will throw a wrench in the works. Meet the pistol squat.

Pistol squats are deceptively difficult, but they are incredibly effective at strengthening the quadriceps, hamstrings, glutes, hip flexors and calf muscles. They also target the core muscles. Not many people realize this at first, but the amount of core activation needed to keep you balanced means this exercise helps to strengthen your mid-region as well as your lower body. It often takes people some time to work up the strength, balance and flexibility to complete this exercise, but it is one of the most effective lower-body workouts around.

Pistol squats are great for improving your overall balance, body awareness and correcting muscle imbalances. When you perform exercises involving both your legs equally, such as the standard squat, one side can take over and take more of the weight of your body. However, this exercise forces one leg to take the full weight of your body, allowing each side to develop an equal amount of strength and balance, eradicating any muscle imbalances you previously had.

Technique

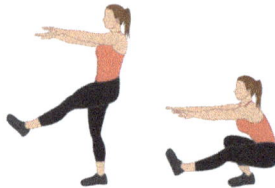

In most cases, this isn't an exercise you can jump straight into and perform correctly the first time. It is essential to develop the mobility in both your legs by gradually building up towards a full pistol squat, and the best way to do this is to follow the progression of exercises below. You can start at the step you feel is most appropriate for you and you can build up this exercise as far as you want.

Beginner (Basic Squat) – Being able to perform a squat is the first step towards developing the mobility needed to perform a pistol squat. Stand with both your feet shoulder-width apart and bend your knees until your thighs are parallel to the ground. Keep your back straight throughout the whole exercise and don't let your knees pass further forward than the line of your toes. Hold this position for a few seconds then raise yourself back up to the starting position.

Intermediate (Chair Pistol) – Now the mobility has been developed, it is time to develop the strength and balance required. Grab a chair, bench or other similar household item and place it behind you. Lift one leg straight out in front of you, bend your other knee and slowly lower yourself down onto the chair. Then lift yourself back up from the seated position using just one leg.

Advanced (Assisted Pistol) – Once you are confident with the chair pistol, you can move on to performing a modified pistol squat with the assistance of a vertical object such as a railing, bannister or pole. Stand in front of the object and place both your hands on either side of it. Lift one leg out in front of you, bend your other knee and lower your body down to the ground, moving your hands down the object to help keep you balanced. Hold this position for a few seconds then raise yourself back up to your starting position.

Expert (Pistol Squat) – Once you have mastered the other stages, you are ready to perform the full pistol squat. Start by standing with your feet together and your arms out straight in front of you. Lift one of your legs straight out in front of you, holding your body weight with the foot that is still on the ground, bend your knee and slowly lower your body down to the ground as far as you can comfortably go. Hold this position for a few seconds then slowly lift yourself back up again without lowering the raised leg. Repeat this movement using the other leg.

9

CARDIO EXERCISES

C ardio training is something that can divide people. Some people are avid runners, enthusiastically signing up for every marathon they can, while others grimace at the thought of running on a treadmill. Regardless of what your fitness goals are, it is beneficial to include cardio in your workouts. However, you don't need to set aside countless hours during the week to improve your cardiovascular fitness. How can this be? The solution is high-intensity interval training (HIIT).

HIIT was recently voted as one of the best fitness methods in a survey conducted by the American College of Sports Medicine, and its popularity continues to grow. This is because it allows you to burn a lot of calories and crank up your heart rate in a much shorter period of time than moderate cardio like jogging or swimming.

But what is HIIT? HIIT involves alternating between bursts of intense exercise followed by lower intensity exercise or complete rest periods. There are a variety of different types of HIIT you can do. For example, bodyweight HIIT (which is the type you will be doing in this book) is where you perform a bodyweight exercise for a short period and then rest in between each exercise. There is also sprint HIIT, where you alternate between running as fast as you can with periods of slow jogging/walking.

Regardless of what type of HIIT workout you do, the most important aspect is the intensity of your workout. You don't need to be going 100%, but you should be working hard enough to the point where you can't comfortably hold a conversation with someone. There are numerous benefits of HIIT, and the exercises in this book, which double as both strength and cardio training, will help you see them.

BENEFITS OF HIIT

Research has shown that HIIT is one of the best and most efficient methods to burn calories and fat compared to moderate cardio. It also causes your body to experience a phenomenon known as excess post-exercise oxygen consumption (EPOC), also known as the 'afterburn' effect. As your body is working intensely, it pushes its repair cycle into overdrive to return the body to its normal physiological state. This means that your body burns calories and fat for hours, even after you have stopped exercising. You can burn more calories and fat with a 15-minute HIIT workout than you can by running on a treadmill for an hour. HIIT is perfect for individuals with busy schedules as you can easily fit these workouts into your day.

When it comes to your health, HIIT works wonders on your body. It improves your cardiovascular health by strengthening your heart muscles, allowing them to pump blood more efficiently, and it can help keep your arteries unclogged by raising your HDL cholesterol (the "good" cholesterol) and lowering your LDL cholesterol (the "bad" cholesterol). It also helps to stabilise blood sugar levels and helps individuals to lose weight and maintain their weight at healthy levels. Overall, it can help reduce the risk of developing diabetes, obesity and high blood pressure, which are sadly on the rise.

Finally, it can help improve your sleep quality, strengthen your immune system and the endorphins that are released can help improve your mental health.

———

HIGH KNEES WITH PAUSE

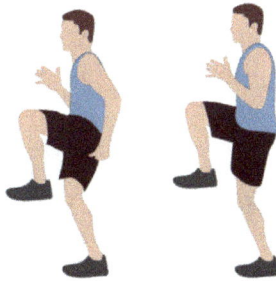

This exercise is a variation of the basic high knees exercise. Stand with your feet about shoulder-width apart, raise your left forearm and lift your right knee up to hip height. From here, engage your core and quickly switch your body position, so your right forearm is raised, and your left knee is up at hip height. Perform 5 repetitions before pausing and holding your raised leg in the air for a few seconds. Repeat this movement, alternating which leg is held up each time.

———

SQUAT JACKS

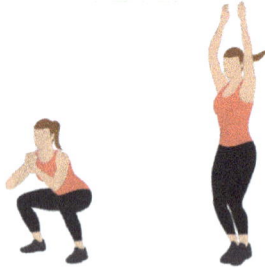

This exercise is the love child of jumping jacks and squats. Squat jacks target the muscles in your lower body whilst cranking up your heart rate and burning lots of calories.

To perform squat jacks, stand with your feet together and arms by your side. Jump into the air and land with your feet spread hip-width apart, dropping into a squat position. Keep your back straight, engage your core and aim to bend your knees until your thighs are parallel to the ground while ensuring your knees don't roll further forward than the line of your toes. From here, drive through your heels and jump back into the air, bringing your feet back in together and raising your arms above your head before landing back in the squat position.

———

ICE SKATERS

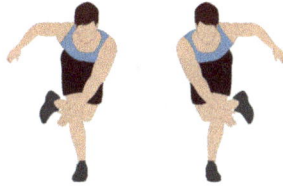

This is an explosive cardio exercise that targets your core, glutes, quads and hamstrings. It also helps to improve your balance and the stability of your hips, knees and ankles.

To perform ice skaters, stand with your feet about shoulder-width apart with your arms by your side. Jump to the right, balance on your right leg and lift your left leg off the ground and cross it behind your body. As you do this movement, bend forward and try to touch the ground with your left hand whilst keeping your left foot off the ground. From here, drive through your right foot and jump to the left, landing on your left foot. Balance on your left leg, cross your right leg behind you while simultaneously bending forward to try and touch the ground with your right hand. Make sure to keep your core engaged, your back straight and look forward as you perform this movement.

If you are just starting, try a little hop as you switch from left to right instead of a big jump. This will help develop your balance and stability. As time goes on, you can focus on being more explosive by jumping further and quickly alternating from left to right.

———

MOUNTAIN CLIMBERS

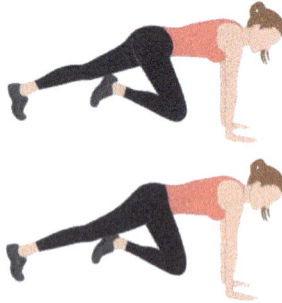

Mountain climbers (which is sometimes referred to as the running plank) is an effective cardio exercise that will also target your core, glutes, legs, arms and shoulder muscles.

To perform this exercise, get into a high plank position with your arms shoulder-width apart and your legs extended out behind you; you want to have a nice straight line from your head to your heels. Keep your back straight, engage your core and keep your wrists directly below your shoulders. Pull your right knee up to your chest then straighten your right leg out behind you again. Then pull your left knee up to your chest and straighten it out behind you again. Continue this movement by alternating between your left and right legs.

When it comes to speed, you don't want to go too fast as you could lose your form and it won't be effectively strengthening your muscles. It is much better to move your legs in a marching movement, really focusing on pulling your knees up to your chest.

———

10

NUTRITION

While exercise is essential for living healthier and working toward your dream body, it is only one part of the many cogs that are essential for maintaining a well-oiled machine. One of the other key components is the healthy fuel you provide your body with and how regularly you feed it.

Now, this does not mean you are restricted to eating only salads for every meal of the day, or you're never allowed to treat yourself. It is more about adding in healthy foods to your diet, rather than cutting out all the things you enjoy.

START THE DAY CORRECTLY

Breakfast is one of the most important meals of the day, yet it is the meal that people have the least. Research has shown that those who regularly eat breakfast are less likely to be obese, develop diabetes and suffer from cardiovascular disease. A high-quality breakfast replenishes your blood sugars and ensures your body is sufficiently fueled up, ready to tackle the day. Breakfast is crucial for days when you plan to do exercise.

However, what you eat for breakfast is important, and lots of people are eating the wrong things. Simple carbohydrates like the ones found in breakfast cereals are often the go-to, but these won't keep you going for long. The more complex the carbohydrate, the more it will fuel you up. Including complex carbohydrates and protein-rich food as part of your breakfast will help you feel fuller for longer and give you more energy for the day.

Here are some examples of healthy foods you can have for breakfast:

- Whole-grain bread with an egg or peanut butter as your source of protein
- If you want to have cereal, avoid standard sugar-loaded breakfast cereals and opt more for whole-grain cereals which are higher in fiber such as muesli, granola and oat bran, add in some fiber-rich fruit such as berries and bananas, and have some milk, yoghurt or chopped nuts as sources of protein

DON'T CUT OUT CARBS

Carbohydrates have quite a bad reputation and are often fully excluded in many different diets. However, your body uses carbohydrates as its main source of energy, especially when you exercise.

Again, the type of carbohydrates you have is important. Carbohydrates are made up of sugar, starch and fiber. Sugars are simple carbohydrates and are commonly found in fizzy drinks, sweets, and as previously mentioned, breakfast cereals. On the other hand, fiber and starch are both complex carbohydrates and are commonly found in whole-grain pasta, whole-grain bread, potatoes and brown rice. Complex carbohydrates are digested much slower than simple carbohydrates, and as a result, they leave us feeling fuller for longer.

Including complex carbohydrates in your diet is vital and can help ensure you maintain a healthy weight and keep your blood sugar levels stable, reducing your chances of developing type 2 diabetes and heart disease. Don't cut out those carbs.

DON'T FORGET PROTEIN

Protein is an essential macronutrient that the body needs to function. Without it, life as we know it wouldn't exist.

Proteins are the building blocks in our body, and they are made up of amino acids. We use them to build and repair our muscles, skin and tendons, as well as use them to make hormones, enzymes, neurotransmitters and red blood cells. Our bodies can also break down protein to use as a source of energy if our carbohydrate stores are low.

Our body can naturally produce certain amino acids, but some can only be found in the food we eat. The amino acids we get via our diet are known as essential amino acids.

The recommendation is that adults have around 0.8 grams of protein per kilogram of body weight (0.36 grams per pound of body weight). If you want to build muscle, the recommendation is that you have around 2.2 grams of protein per kilogram of body weight (1 gram of protein per pound of body weight).

When it comes to sources of protein, generally animal protein such as poultry, red meat and fish contain all the essential amino acids the body needs. If you don't eat meat, you can also get protein from eggs, dairy products such as milk and yoghurt, and plant-based sources such as beans and lentils. You want to focus more on lean proteins that have low levels of saturated and trans fats, as well as keeping your red and processed meat consumption to a minimum.

NOT ALL FATS ARE BAD

Fats are often avoided as they are seen as harmful for our body. Although this is correct about specific types of fat, this isn't the case for all of them. Some fats are actually good for you and help to enhance your overall health. It is important to know which fats are good for you and which fats you should avoid.

When it comes to the different types of fats, the two types that are the most harmful are saturated and trans fats. Try to avoid trans fats and only ingest saturated fats in moderation. Any fats that are solid in form at room temperature tend to contain saturated fats. Examples include high-fat dairy foods (butter and sour cream), tropical oils (palm oil, coconut oil and cocoa butter) and practically all animal fats (except for fish fat). Trans fats can commonly be found in fried food, baked goods and processed foods. Ingesting too much of these fats can increase your LDL cholesterol levels.

Cholesterol is a type of fat in the blood, and you have two different forms: low-density lipoprotein (LDL) and high-density lipoprotein (HDL). LDL is commonly referred to as "bad" cholesterol and increases your risk of heart disease if you have high levels in your blood. On the other hand, HDL is commonly referred to as "good" cholesterol, as it travels through your blood, picking up other types of cholesterol and taking them to the liver to be broken down. Research has shown that high levels of HDL cholesterol can help lower the risk of having a stroke or heart attack.

The two types of fat that are good for you are monounsaturated and polyunsaturated fats. Both these types of fats can help decrease LDL cholesterol levels and reduce your risk of developing heart disease in the future. These fats tend to be in liquid form at room temperature. Some great sources of monounsaturated fats include nuts (cashews, pecans and almonds), vegetable oils (olive oil), avocado and peanut butter. You can find polyunsaturated fats in many plant-based foods and oils. Notably, omega-3 fatty acids are a type of polyunsaturated fat and can commonly be found in different types of oily fish such as salmon, trout and sardines.

Make sure to focus on including the healthy types of fat and avoiding the unhealthy types as much as possible.

FRUIT AND VEGETABLES

We all know that fruit and vegetables are extremely healthy to eat. They're full of fiber, vitamins and minerals, and have low amounts of fat and calories. There are so many different varieties too, so you are bound to find some you like.

Eating a variety of fruit and vegetables will help ensure you are providing your body with a wide range of vitamins, minerals and antioxidants, and an easy way to accomplish this is to try and "eat the rainbow" (sadly I am not talking about Skittles). Include fruit and vegetables of various colours and try to fill half your plate with them at each meal.

REGULAR MEALTIMES

As important as it is to eat enough carbohydrates, proteins and fat, a lot of people fail to focus on one of the most important features of a healthy diet: regular mealtimes.

It is very easy to skip breakfast if you have overslept or avoid lunch if you are bogged down with work. Some people even deliberately skip meals as a way to cut out calories in an attempt to lose weight. However, skipping meals can significantly affect your energy levels and cause you to snack, overeat or binge on less healthy foods.

Contrary to popular belief, research has shown that eating more regular meals throughout the day can actually help you lose weight and maintain healthy cholesterol and insulin levels. It can also keep your energy levels high, minimize cravings and keep you feeling fuller for longer. The key is to keep your mealtimes consistent, aiming to eat every 3 to 4 hours.

WHAT TO EAT BEFORE AND AFTER A WORKOUT

It is important to fuel your body up with the right food and fluids before, during and after you exercise to help keep your blood sugar levels high, perform at the highest possible level and recover in a shorter period of time. There isn't a strict guide to follow when it comes to this, but it is beneficial to know what to eat when it comes to your workout.

If you have a few hours before your workout, make sure you are drinking sufficient fluids and are consuming healthy carbohydrates like whole-grain pasta, whole-grain toast and fruits and vegetables. Try to avoid saturated fats and protein because they take longer to digest, redirecting oxygen and blood to the stomach rather than to the muscles. If you have less time before your workout, aim to have some fruit.

Make sure you are keeping hydrated and having small sips of fluids frequently throughout your exercise routine. Unless you are exercising at a high intensity for over an hour, you don't need to worry about eating during your workout.

After you have finished exercising, you want to top up the tank. As you have used carbohydrates as your primary source of energy during your workout, you need to replenish your stores around 20 to 60 minutes after you have finished. Also, make sure to have some protein after your workout to help repair your muscles and allow them to grow.

This is a rough outline of the nutrition you need when it comes to exercising, but everyone is different. Your body will require different nutrition depending on the type of exercise you have done. Never forget that the food you put into your body is just as crucial as the exercise you are doing.

TREAT YOURSELF

This is potentially one of the most important things to remember. There are plenty of things we can do to eat healthier and plenty of foods we should probably avoid having. However, there is absolutely nothing wrong with a treat now and again. If you are at your spouse's birthday celebrations and you fancy a slice of cake and a glass of prosecco, absolutely go for it. You enjoy that cake! There is no point making yourself miserable by cutting out all of the "unhealthy" foods you love. With anything in life, the key is moderation.

SAMPLES OF WEEKLY WORKOUT AND MEAL PLANS

The workout routines in this book are different from other exercise programs. Instead of focusing on completing a set number of repetitions of an exercise, the aim is to complete as many repetitions of that exercise as possible in a set period of time. The reason for this is because everyone is different. If everyone has to perform 10 push-ups, some individuals may be able to do them without breaking a sweat, whereas others may struggle to do two or three, causing them to feel deflated if they can't reach the target. This method is a much more positive and effective way to train. Your only competition is who you were yesterday. You can exercise at your own pace and go faster or slower depending on your fitness levels. The routines will only take around 20 to 30 minutes to complete, making them very easy to fit into your day.

In the beginning stages, you may only be able to perform a few repetitions of the exercises, and there is absolutely nothing wrong with that. Everyone has to start somewhere, and the more you practice, the more your strength will develop, and the more repetitions you will be able to do. It is important to keep track of the number of repetitions that you perform as this is a great way to track your progress.

If you are just starting, limit your workouts to three days a week and ensure you take adequate rest days in between. On the days that you are resting, it can be beneficial to do some light cardio like jogging, swimming or even skipping. This isn't essential, but the light cardio will help increase your heart rate, increasing the blood flow to the muscles and providing them with more nutrients to help them repair quicker. DOMS can be an issue for those starting as their bodies aren't used to this new level of physical activity. Fortunately, the effects of DOMS lessen as time goes on and your body adjusts.

As you become fitter, you will find the amount of exercise you're currently doing will get easier. When you feel like this, it is time to apply the key principles you learned about in Chapter 1 and progressively overload your body, and there are several ways you can do this. You can increase the frequency (working out four times a week instead of three), the intensity (adding in more exercises to each round or increasing the number of rounds you do) or the duration of your workout (working for 60 seconds instead of 45 seconds)

When you are working out, try not to rest for too long between each exercise as your muscles will start to cool down and stiffen. Limit your rest period between each exercise from 30 seconds up to 1 minute. Once you have completed a round of exercises, give yourself 2 to 3 minutes of rest before starting again.

The beauty of these routines is that they can be individually adapted to suit your personal preferences. Some people prefer to train the whole body at once while others like to target specific muscle groups on certain days, and examples of each have been included in this chapter. There is no set way to work out, and it is entirely up to you which method you choose to do.

TARGETED MUSCLE GROUP PLAN (EXAMPLE)

Monday (Back and Arms): 2 rounds of exercises - 45 seconds per exercise + 30 seconds rest in between exercises. 2 minutes rest between each round.

- Warm-up – mini cardio and dynamic upper body stretches
- Push-ups
- Wide overhand pull-up (if you have a bar) or overhand inverted row (if you don't have a bar)
- Back widows
- Underhand chin-up (if you have a bar) or underhand inverted row (if you don't have a bar)
- Crab walk
- Dolphin kicks
- Tricep dips
- Cool down – slow walk/jog for 2-3 minutes and static upper body stretches

Tuesday: Rest

Wednesday (Chest, Shoulders and Core): 2 rounds of exercises - 45 seconds per exercise + 30 seconds rest in between exercises. 2 minutes rest between each round.

- Warm-up – mini cardio and dynamic upper body stretches
- Wide push-up
- Lateral deltoid flies
- Internal rotations with left shoulder
- Internal rotation with right shoulder
- Drunken mountain climbers
- Burpees
- Seated ab circles to the left
- Seated ab circles to the right
- Cool-down – slow walk/jog for 2-3 minutes and static upper

body stretches

Thursday: Rest

Friday (Glutes, Legs and Cardio): 2 rounds of exercises - 45 seconds per exercise + 30 seconds rest in between exercises. 2 minutes rest between each round.

- Warm-up – mini cardio and dynamic lower body stretches
- Slick floor bridge curls
- Hip thrusts
- Squat jacks
- Single leg calf raises with right leg
- Single leg calf raises with left leg
- Side leg raise with right leg
- Side leg raise with left leg
- Split squat jump
- Cool-down – slow walk/jog for 2-3 minutes and static lower body stretches

Saturday: Rest day

Sunday: Rest day

FULL BODY WORKOUT PLAN (EXAMPLE)

Monday: Rest day

Tuesday: 2 rounds of exercises - 45 seconds per exercise + 30 seconds rest in between exercises. 2 minutes rest between each round.

- Warm-up – mini cardio and dynamic stretches
- Decline push-up
- Full bow
- Superman
- Spiderman push-up

- Scissor kicks
- Ice skaters
- Bulgarian split squat with right leg
- Bulgarian split squat with left leg
- Squats
- Cool-down – slow walk/jog for 2-3 minutes and static stretches

Wednesday: Rest day

Thursday: 2 rounds of exercises - 45 seconds per exercise + 30 seconds rest in between exercises. 2 minutes rest between each round.

- Warm-up – mini cardio and dynamic stretches
- Clap push-up
- Shadowboxing
- Bicep curls
- Launch squats
- Scapular push-up
- Mountain climbers
- Reverse plank
- Single-leg glute bridge with right leg
- Single-leg glute bridge with left leg
- Cool-down – slow walk/jog for 2-3 minutes and static stretches

Friday: Rest day

Saturday: Rest day

Sunday: 2 rounds of exercises - 45 seconds per exercise + 30 seconds rest in between exercises. 2 minutes rest between each round.

- Warm-up – mini cardio and dynamic stretches
- Burpees

- Squat jacks
- Incline push-up
- Split squat jump
- Handstand push-up (or any of the progressions)
- Wide overhand pull-up (if you have a bar) or overhand inverted row (if you don't have a bar)
- Side leg raise with right leg
- Side leg raise with left leg
- Sumo squats
- Cool-down – slow walk/jog for 2-3 minutes and static stretches

If you would like 4 weeks' worth of routines, make sure to download your essential fitness bundle mentioned at the front and back of the book.

MEAL PLAN (EXAMPLE)

There are a variety of healthy foods that you can put into your body to help boost your metabolism. Alternating the types of foods that you consume will help to prevent boredom and reduce the chance of you falling into unhealthy eating habits.

The example of the meal plan below will incorporate the basic food groups that you should have daily, and you can modify it as you please.

- Breakfast: 2 poached eggs, 1 slice of whole-grain toast, and 2 rashers of fat-free bacon.
- Mid-morning snack: 1 cup of fat-free yoghurt, a sliced banana, and a handful of blueberries.
- Lunch: Avocado, pesto and mozzarella wraps
- Mid-afternoon snack: 1 tablespoon of peanut butter on a slice of whole-grain toast.
- Dinner: Chicken stir-fry with egg noodles, broccoli, carrots

and baby corn.
- Dessert – Ice cream with strawberries

Everyone has different dietary requirements and preferences, so this is merely an illustration of the types of delicious and filling food you can have throughout the day. Remember, healthy food does not need to be bland; it can be some of the best-tasting food you will ever have.

Enjoy exercising and enjoy healthy eating. Your body will thank you for it.

CONCLUSION

There are always obstacles that prevent us from exercising, and life has a knack for getting in the way. Sometimes it feels like there are not enough hours in the day to fit in everything we want to do. However, you've taken the first step in a life-changing journey by reading this book. You have realized that living healthier and achieving your dream body does not have to cost you a fortune; you don't need to take large chunks out of your bank account each month to pay for expensive gym memberships or personal trainers. It can be achieved at home.

The bodyweight exercises that you have learned about in this book are exercises that you will be able to do anywhere and at any time. You now have a greater understanding of the anatomy of the muscles in your body, and you now know which exercises you can do to train them effectively. You also know about the importance of nutrition and healthy eating. If you keep to regular mealtimes and add in more healthy components to your diet, while still enjoying the other foods you like, you will start to shed pounds gradually and safely. Regular exercise will also boost your metabolism and that is why it is so important to combine these two steps for optimal results. Regular exercise and healthy eating independently boost your metabolism and they are incredibly effective when they are combined.

There's no better time than now to start exercising more. However, don't forget that this is a (hypothetical) marathon and not a sprint; change doesn't happen overnight. Working towards your dream body does take a lot of hard work and determination, and sadly there are no short cuts. Fortunately, with this book, you have everything you need to get there, and you are more than capable of achieving your goals.

Remember the basics, and don't forget to warm up before and cool down after your workout. They may add a few minutes to your routine, but they are essential to help avoid any injuries occurring and help to prevent you from experiencing any pain or stiffness during or after your workout. Don't forget to update your exercise routine when it starts getting easier by gradually changing the frequency, intensity or duration. Listen to your body and remember to stay within your limits. As you get stronger and fitter, you will be able to perform more repetitions and attempt more advanced exercises.

Keep on pushing yourself. Remember, your only competition is the person you were yesterday. Best of luck! You got this!

'Exercise is king. Nutrition is queen. Put them together and you've got a kingdom'

— JACK LALANNE

DON'T FORGET YOUR FREE GIFT!

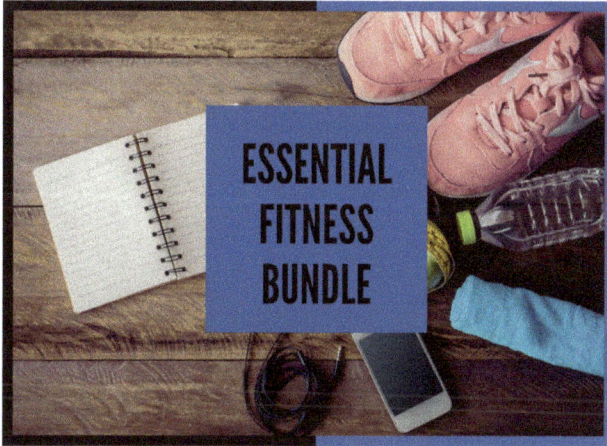

As a thank you for purchasing this book, I have thrown in a special gift for you. This bundle includes:

- An essential fitness checklist to ensure you have everything you need for your workout and where you can buy them for a great price
- 4 weeks' worth of exercise routines
- Two different types of personalisable fitness diary and a progress tracker to help you monitor your progress and track your success
- A weekly meal planner to help you organise what you'll be eating each day

The last thing I want is for your hard work to go to waste because you do not have the essentials. To receive your bundle, visit the link:

https://agscott.activehosted.com/f/1

ACKNOWLEDGEMENTS

If you had told me that 2020 would be the year I start writing books, I would have thought you were crazy. I truly am not the typical "writer" type, but hey, it's funny how things work out and where life takes you. I have truly loved writing this book, but it has been much harder than I ever thought it would be. However, it has also been one of the most rewarding things I have ever done, and I have learned so much during this process. Truth be told, I didn't go through this alone, and I couldn't have written this book without the support of some wonderful people.

Firstly, I would like to thank my incredible mother, Eleanor. Words can't describe how grateful I am for everything you have ever done for me; I wouldn't be the man I am today if it wasn't for your constant love and support. Your continued enthusiasm, volunteering to read through the book, the thousands of cups of tea you made me, and even being the tester of all the exercises in the book have all been instrumental during this process. The book wouldn't have been possible without you.

To my wonderful girlfriend, Millie. You have been involved in this book more than you will ever know. From volunteering to read early drafts and helping with cover designs (and even designing your own), to your immense patience in putting up with my constant talk about the book. Thank you so much for your support with everything I do. I promise I'll give you some time off before asking you to read over any more book drafts because you truly deserve it. Thank you for all the love and the memories.

I would like to say a massive thank you to Dr Oliver Jones, founder of TeachMeAnatomy.info, for allowing me to use some of his anatomy diagrams in my book and for the high-quality information on his website. The images and your website have been invaluable for both the book and my time at medical school by making the complexities of the human body much easier to understand. You have truly helped make anatomy more understandable for medical students all across the world, and I can safely say on everyone's behalf, we are truly grateful.

To my sister, Jenna. I am extremely grateful for the constant support you have given me over the years and the thousands of free haircuts. You have always had an amazing way of seeing the positives in every situation, and that mindset has been something I have tried to carry with me in everything I do. We have had some incredible memories and laughs, and I am unbelievably proud of everything you have achieved.

To Tom. You have been a fantastic father figure for me. You have taught me so much over the years, and I am extremely thankful for how well you have cared for my mother and me. You have shown me the type of father I want to be when I am older, and I am so appreciative for you coming into my life.

Last but certainly not least, I would like to say a massive thank you to the rest of my family and my friends from home, university and overseas. There are too many of you to name but you know who you are. You have given me so many incredible memories, experiences and laughs over the years, and I am grateful to have met every single one of you.

REFERENCES

Active, E. (2020). *10 Fantastic Home Chest Workouts to Try.* Home Workouts & Health. www. everyoneactive.com.

American Heart Association. (2015). *Food as Fuel Before, During and After Workouts.* www.heart.org

Anderson, C. (2020). *8 Benefits of High-Intensity Interval Training (HIIT).* www.shape.com

Anna. (2018). *7 Easy Warm Up Exercises For Sensitive Wrists.* www.fitnclassy.org

Bailey, A. (2019). *What Muscles Does the Mountain Climber Exercise Work?* www.livestrong.com

Belluz, J. (2019). *How to get the most out of your exercise time, according to science.* www.vox.com

Boldt, A. (2017). *The Importance of Working Out Your Legs.* www.livestrong.com

Boly, J. (2019). *Why the Hip Thrust Is a Fantastic Tool for Building and Powerful Glutes.* www.bar-bend.com

Boly, J. (2020). *The Bulgarian Split Squat Is The Ultimate Leg Builder.* www.barbend.com

Brenner-Roach, T. (2020). *How to Warm Up for Bodyweight Exercises.* www.liftlearngrow.com

Bruno, B. (2013). *Hamstring Hell: Sliding Leg Curls.* www.t-nation.com

Calvert, M. Samuel, E. (2020). *These 13 HIIT Workouts Will Make You Forget Boring Cardio.* www.-menshealth.com

Cavaliere, J. (2016). *Home Back Workout (No Pullup Bar!).* www.athleanx.com

Cavaliere, J. (2017). *How NOT to swing on Hanging Ab Exercises.* www.athleanx.com

Cavaliere, J. (2018). *Hanging Leg Raise | How-To.* www.athleanx.com

Cavaliere, J. (2018). *Intense Ab Workout | 7 Minutes (FOLLOW ALONG).* www.athleanx.com

Cavaliere, J. (2019). *The Official Pull-Up Checklist (AVOID MISTAKES).* www.athleanx.com

Cavaliere, J. (2020). *The PERFECT Home Workout (Sets and Reps included)*. www.athleanx.com

Chandler, S. (2019). *What Are the 3 Main Hip Flexor Muscles?* www.livestrong.com

Chertoff, J. (2019). *Pylo Push-ups: What Are the Benefits and How to Master This Move*. www.healthline.com

Chertoff, J. (2019). *The Benefits of Dynamic Stretching and How to Get Started*. www.healthline.com

Coachmag. (2019). *How To Do Triceps Dips*. Exercises. www.coachmag.co.uk

Cooper, E. (2020) *Home Arms Workout: 7 Bodyweight Moves to Build Bigger Arms When You're Stuck Indoors*. www.menshealth.com.

Costa, P.B. Baptista, H. Fukuda, D.H. (2011). *Warm-up, Stretching, and Cool-down Strategies for Combat Sports*. Strength and Conditioning Journal. 33(6): 71-79.

Cronkleton, E. (2019). *16 Cooldown Exercises You Can Do After Any Workout*. www.healthline.com

Cronkleton, E. (2019). *The Benefits of Wide Push-ups and How to Do Them*. www.healthline.com

Dale, P. (2020). *Hyperextension Guide – Muscles Worked, Variations And Benefits*. www.fitnessvolt.com

Davis, N. (2019). *How to Do a Bulgarian Split Squat the Right Way*. www.healthline.com

Dewar, M. (2018). *Jumping Lunges – Muscles Worked, Exercise Demo, and Benefits*. www.barbend.com

Doctorjeal. (2020). *Why it it called a burpee?* Health & Fitness. www.doctorjeal.com

Donatelli, R. (2020). *What is The Core?* www.sportsmd.com

Eastnine. (2019). *Five Principles Of Training*. www.eastnine.fit.

Edgely, R. (2019). *How to Get More From Your Bicep Curls*. www.menshealth.com

Exercisegoals.com. (2020). *Rotator Cuff Exercises – Rotator Cuff Strengthening Exercises*. www.exercisegoals.com

Familydoctor.org. (2017). *Hydration for Athletes*. www.familydoctor.org.

Fanslau, J. (2016). *The Shadowboxing Workout That Will Leave You a Sweaty Mess*. www.menshealth.com

Fernandes, T.L. Pedrinelli, A. Hernandez, A.J. (2011). *Muscle Injury - Physiopathology, Diagnosis, Treatment, and Clinical Presentation*. US National Library of Medicine. NCBI. 46(3): 247–255.

Fisher, K. (2019). *Body Water Percentage: Average, Ideal, How To Maintain And Determine*. WebMD.

Fit Father Project. (2018). *One Leg Calf Raises (GET BIGGER CALVES TODAY!)*. www.fitfatherproject.com

Gales, M. (2015). How to Throw a Jab *(A step by step guide for Beginners)*. www.youtube.com/EverlastNutritionFitnessiswithin

Gales, M. (2015). *How to throw a Cross in boxing (A step by step guide for Beginners)*. www.youtube.com/EverlastNutritionFitnessiswithin

Gales, M. (2015). *How to Throw a Hook in Boxing (A step by step guide for Beginners)*. www.youtube.com/EverlastNutritionFitnessiswithin

Gales, M. (2015). *How to Throw an Uppercut – Boxing (A step by step guide for Beginners).* www.youtube.com/EverlastNutritionFitnessiswithin

Garage Gym Power. (2020). *No Bar? No Problem! Check Out These 9 Pull-Up Alternatives For Home.* www.*garagegympower*.com

Get Healthy U (2020). *How To Do Skaters.* www.gethealthyu.com

Get Strong. (2016). *All About Scap Pushups.* www.getstrong.fit

Get Strong. (2017). *Lunge Kicks Exercise Guide.* www.getstrong.fit

Grand, T. (2014). *5 Surprising Benefits of Training Your Glutes.* www.inspiyr.com

Gunnars, K. (2018). *Protein Intake – How Much Protein Should You Eat Per Day?*

Hall, B. (2019). *The Reverse Plank is the Best Core Exercise You're Not Doing.* www.stack.com

Harlan, T. Coursealt, J. (2020). *Exercise How To: Superman.* www.drgourmet.com

Hanson, C. (2018). *The Importance of Hydration During Exercise: Fighting the Thirst Curse.* *www.progenex.com*

Harris-Fry, N. (2019). *How To Do A Dumbbell Shoulder Press.* www.coachmag.co.uk

Harris-Fry, N. Snape, J. (2019). *The Lateral Raise: How To Do It And Five Top Form Tips.* www.coachmag.co.uk

Harvard Health Publishing. (2020). *Eating Frequency and Weight Loss.* Healthbeat. www.health.harvard.edu

Harvard Health Publishing. (2020). *The real-world benefits of strengthening your core.* Healthbeat. www.health.harvard.edu

Higuera, V. (2018). *Medial Epicondylitis (Golfer's Elbow).* www.healthline.com

Issa. (2020). *Understanding and Using the Overload Principle.* www.issaonline.com.

Joint Ventures. (2016). *Which Are My Core Muscles?* www.jointventurespt.com

Johnson, J. (2020). *Bulgarian Split Squats Vs. Split Squats.* www.healthyliving.azcentral.com

Jones, O. (2017). *Muscles of the Pectoral Region.* www.teachmeanatomy.info

Jones, O. (2020) *Muscles in the Posterior Compartment of the Leg.* www.teachmeanatomy.info

Jones, O. (2020). *Muscles of the Gluteal Region.* www.teachmeanatomy.info

Jones, O. (2020). *Muscles in the Medial Compartment of the Thigh.* www.teachmeanatomy.info

Jones, O. (2020). *The Intrinsic Muscles of the Shoulder.* www.teachmeanatomy.info

Jones, O. (2020). *The Superficial Back Muscles.* www.teachmeanatomy.info

Kastner, J. (2020). *What Muscles Do Deltoid Flies Work?* Fitness. www.livestrong.com

Kester, S. (2019). *How to Do Side Leg Raises Two Ways.* www.healthline.com

Khatri, M. (2019.) *What is Dehydration? What Causes It?* WebMD.

Kilroy, D. (2019). *Eating the Right Foods for Exercise.* www.healthline.com

Lindberg, S. (2019). *How to Do Scissor Kicks.* www.healthline.com

Lindberg, S. (2019). *How to Do Wide Grip Pullups.* www.healthline.com

Lindberg, S. (2019). *7 Benefits of Doing Squats and Variations to Try.*

Madbarz. (2016). *Incline VS Decline Push-ups: What's The Difference?* www.madbarz.com

Madbarz. (2017). *Why Clap Push Ups Maximise Your Chest Growth And How To Do Them.* www.madbarz.com

Madell, R. Nall, R. (2019). *Good Fats, Bad Fats, and Heart Disease.* www.healthline.com

Malone, M. (2019). *What Muscles Do Burpees Work?* www.livestrong.com

Marcin, A. (2019). *How to Do Chair Dips.* www.healthline.com

Marcin, A. (2020). *What Are The Benefits Of Aerobic Exercise?* www.healthline.com

Marengo, K. (2020). *Simple Carbohydrates vs. Complex Carbohydrates.* www.healthline.com

Martin, D. (2020). *Trapezius Muscle: Stiff Neck, Headache, Eye, Jaw, Pain.* www.thewellnessdigest.com

Masters, M. (2016). *Why Your Random Eating Schedule Is Risky For Your Health.* www.health.com

Matthews, M. (2020). *4 Rotator Cuff Exercises That You Should Be Doing (and Why).* www.legionathletics.com

Mayo Clinic. (2017). *Metabolism and weight loss: How you burn calories.* www.mayoclinic.org

Mayo Clinic. (2018). *HDL Cholesterol: How to boost your "good" cholesterol.* www.mayoclinic.org

Mazzo, L. (2019). *The Sumo Squat Is the Best Squat Exercise for Your Lower Thighs.* www.shape.com

Miller, J. (2020). *The Reverse Hyper.* www.powerliftingbelts.org

Monica, S. (2020). *The Art of Shadowboxing | Why we Shadowbox.* www.gloveworx.com

Mortazavi, T. (2020). *7 Benefits of Having Strong Legs.* www.allwomenstalk.com

Mulkerrins, I. (2019). *The importance of regular meal times.* www.itsahealthylifestyle.org

Munye, A. (2020). *Wide Grip Pull-Ups – How To Do, Muscles Worked & Benefits.* www.ammfitness.co.uk

Nestler, P. (2017). *Hip Abductions... You're Doing It WRONG.* www.youtube.com/CoachPJNestler

Ng, N. (2019). *How To Do A Dumbbell Fly.* www.livestrong.com

Nguyen, J. (2010). *7 Basic Boxing Combinations.* www.expertboxing.com

Nick. (2017). *How To Build Strong Legs (And Why It's Important).* www.integrativeoesteopathy.com.au

Nick. (2018). *How To Build A Strong Back (And Why It's Important).* www.integrativeosteopathy.com.au

Osterweil, N. (2020). *The Benefits of Protein.* WedMD

Perry, M. (2019). *Try This 5-Minute Dynamic Stretching Routine to Prep for Any Workout.* www.greatist.com

Petre, A. (2016). *The 17 Best Protein Sources for Vegans and Vegetarians.* www.healthline.com

PumpOne. (2012). *Top 5 Strongest Muscles in the Body.* www.pumpone.com

PureGym. (2020). *How To Do A Shoulder Press.* www.puregym.com

Quinn, E. (2019). *How to Do a Reverse Plank.* www.verywellfit.com

Quinn, E. (2019). *How to Do the Single Leg Bridge.* www.verywellfit.coms

Ratcliffe, J. (2019). *Best Wrap Fillings.* www.olivemagazine.com

Redefining Strength. (2020). *Scapular Push Ups.* www.redefiningstrength.com

Rogers, P. (2020). *How to Do a Hanging Leg Raise.* www.verywellfit.com

Roth, S.M. (2006). *Why Does Lactic Acid Build Up in Muscles? And Why Does It Cause Soreness?* The Body. Scientific American.

Seana. (2015). *Freeletics Exercises: Handstand Push-ups.* www.freeletics.com

Smith, D. (2015). *13 Legit Reasons to Start Bodyweight Training Today.* www.greatist.com

Stryker, K. (2012). *Five Reasons Why Burpees Should Be Your Favorite Exercise.* www.12minuteathlete.com

Stryker, K. (2013). *Handstand Push Ups: Why They Rock (And How To Start Doing Them).* www.12minuteathlete.com

Tavel, R. (2019). *Get Warmed Up With This Dynamic Stretching Routine.* www.menshealth.com

Tapp, T. (2015). *How to Pistol Squat – Beginner Progressions Steps – Tapp Brothers.* www.youtube.com/TappBrothers

Thomason, K. (2019). *How To Do A Squat Jack For A Serious Cardio Workout.* www.womenshealthmag.com

Trifocus Fitness Academy. (2017). *Why Pectoral Strength is Necessary.* www.trifocusfitnessacademy.co.za

Tucker, A. (2020). *A 15-Minute No-Equipment Core Workout You Can Do at Home.* Fitness. www.self.com.

Ultimate Performance. (2020). *How To Fix Your Posture With Strength Training.* www.up-australia.com

Unique Health and Fitness (2019). *Top Benefits Of Having Strong Glutes.* www.uniquehealthandfitness.com

Venuto, T. (2020). *Bodyweight Hip Thrusts: The Next Step In Glute Training.* www.burnthefatinnercircle.com

Waehner, P. (2018). *Why You Need to Work Your Chest Muscles.* www.verywellfit.com

Ward, B. (2018). *5 Amazing Benefits Of The Pistol Squat (#4 Will Make Your Jaw Drop).* www.theworkoutdigest.com

Washmuth, D. (2020). *Pectoralis Minor: Function, Blood Supply and Innervation.* www.study.com.

Weir, J. (2017). *What Muscles Are Worked With Hanging Leg Raises?* www.livestrong.com

Weller, J. (2019). *10 Gym Membership Statistics You Need to Know.* www.glofox.com

Williams, L. (2019). *How to Do Spiderman Pushups.* www.verywellfit.com

Winderl, A.M. (2018). *Here's Exactly How to Do a Push-up Correctly.* Fitness. www.self.com

Winderl, A.M. (2018). *10 Great Stretches to Do After An Upper-Body Workout.* Fitness. www.self.com.

Winderl, A.M. (2018). *10 Great Stretches to Do After A Lower-Body Workout.* Fitness. www.self.com.

Wood, M. (2019). *The Benefits of Arm Exercises: Why You Need a Strong Upper Body.* www.michaelwoodfitness.com.

Yoga Outlet. (2015). *How to Do Downward-Facing Dog in Yoga.* www.yogaoutlet.com

Zelman, K.M. (2019). *Simple Secrets to Healthy Eating and Portion Control.* WebMD.

www.ingramcontent.com/pod-product-compliance
Lightning Source LLC
Chambersburg PA
CBHW050730030426
42336CB00012B/1498